Neurology: What shall I do?

3

Supplied as a service
to medicine
by

GlaxoWellcome

Other titles in this series:

Ophthalmology: What shall I do?
by Jack Kanski and Bev Daily

Paediatrics: What shall I do?
by Mike Liberman and Bev Daily

Neurology

What shall I do?

Second edition

Dafydd Thomas, MA, MD, FRCP

Bev Daily, MB, BS

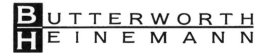

Butterworth-Heinemann
Linacre House, Jordan Hill, Oxford OX2 8DP
A division of Reed Educational and Professional Publishing Ltd

℞ A member of the Reed Elsevier plc group

OXFORD   BOSTON   JOHANNESBURG
MELBOURNE   NEW DELHI   SINGAPORE

First published 1989
Second edition 1996

British Library Cataloguing in Publication Data
A catalogue record for this book is
available from the British Library

Library of Congress Cataloguing in Publication Data
A catalogue record for this book is
available from the Library of Congress

ISBN 0 7506 3195 3

Typesetting by David Gregson Associates, Beccles, Suffolk
Printed in Great Britain by Biddles Ltd, Guildford and King's Lynn

Contents

Contents

Preface

A week in politics may be a long time but seven years in neurology is not. Nevertheless, since 1989, when this book was first published, new treatments have appeared and there have been a number of changes in case management brought about, not least, by the increased availability of scanning. And there may be some exciting developments in the pipeline ...

D.J.T.
B.N.J.D.

Note
The experience of the authors, reflecting the prescribing nuances in the special field of neurology, means that some of the discussion may involve medicines outside of their licensed UK use. The reader is advised to refer to the manufacturer's Data Sheet prior to prescribing.

Preface to the first edition

Neurology: What shall I do? is a book of questions asked by a GP and answered by a consultant neurologist.

In this area of medicine there is often only a very narrow divide between urgent and non-urgent cases. Neurologists are pretty thin on the ground and the difference between an urgent and non-urgent appointment could be the difference between 24 hours and 24 weeks.

The GP, therefore, should be able to sort out those patients who do need a quick referral and those who do not. The paradox is, of course, that this presupposes he or she already knows the diagnosis of the condition for which the opinion is being sought. 'Mr Brown's headache is due to a meningioma – I shall ask for an urgent appointment. Mrs Smith's headache is just a muscular contraction problem – she can wait until January.'

Neurology has the reputation of being a difficult subject mainly because of the way neuroanatomy is taught, in such excruciating detail, at medical school. An esoteric approach, as it happens, to a far from esoteric subject. Thirty per cent of all acute admissions have a neurological element as do most geriatric admissions and virtually all young, chronic sick admissions.

The idea of this book, therefore, is to suggest an approach to some of the neurological problems faced by a GP in his surgery. Ninety-five per cent of neurology is relatively straightforward, if not simple. There is no need for the reader to 'bull up' on the long forgotten relations of the internal capsule or the component parts of the cerebellum.

A large part of the GP's exposure to neurological medicine is a mixture of the diagnostic and the situational. What action should be taken when a child falls from a climbing frame and is stunned for a few seconds? Is it wise to advise a patient with a stiff neck against going to an osteopath? Should an octogenarian Don Juan be taken off his L-dopa? How long should a headache be left before referral is made?

The answers to these questions, and many more, are given by a neurologist. Some of his colleagues may disagree with some of the answers. This book is not, therefore, like many textbooks, intended to be Holy Scripture. Neither does it presume to be comprehensive – most GPs could think of another 100 questions from their own experience with no difficulty.

It is hoped, however, that not only will it give the working GP some idea of what to look for in day-to-day encounters, but also present to the trainer some subject matter with which to torment the trainee. It might also make slightly more street-wise those younger doctors whose experience has not yet led them beyond the hospital wards, the relations of the internal capsule, small print and large textbooks.

The questions have been grouped under broad headings. Particular attention has been placed on the index which uses question number rather than page number so that it provides a quick easy reference even when the patient is sitting in the surgery: 'I'll be with you in a moment, Mr Jones'.

Mention is also made of investigations such as EEG, CT, MRI scan and angiography which are not available to the vast majority of patellar-hammer wielding GPs. It is hoped that this will enable them to do a little bit of judicious forewarning when referral is made: 'You might have told me, Doctor!'

D.J.T.
B.N.J.D.

Epilepsy

Question 1.   'Can I ride my bike, Mum?'

The parents of an 8-year-old boy bring their son to the surgery. He has had three grand mal attacks in the previous 6 months. Idiopathic epilepsy has been diagnosed. He is now on anticonvulsant therapy. He has always been an active child. The parents ask whether he should be allowed to ride his bicycle, ride his pony, do PE at school. What advice would you give?

Children with epilepsy:

- Should not ride a bicycle in traffic.
- Should be able to ride a horse (but not on the road) unless they have poorly controlled major attacks.
- Should not swim without a personal attendant of some kind and should not swim either out of their own depth or their attendant's depth.
- Should be discouraged from exercises involving heights.

Children with epilepsy should be encouraged to lead as normal a life as possible within certain safety limits. This is so that they can develop their personalities in a satisfactory manner without acquiring too many 'chips on their shoulders'.

The type of advice given and the way that certain dangers should be emphasized depends on the personalities of the child and the parents as well as on the type of epilepsy. A child who is a dare-devil with rather careless parents will need checking to avoid physical harm occurring during his episodes, whereas an inhibited somewhat introverted child of over-cautious parents may disappear into his shell completely if he is warned too strongly and such a family will need encouragement rather than caution.

The type of epilepsy is very important. Infrequent major attacks may present less of a problem than more frequent minor episodes, although the parents and the child may not think so. It should be explained to them that a child with petit mal may be getting several episodes an hour and therefore statistically the chances of something going wrong due to a momentary lapse of consciousness and concentration are very much greater than in someone who has one major attack every 6–12 months. Some patients report that their attacks only occur when their mind is idling. Unfortunately, this not totally reassuring because the brain is often idling while cycling and swimming and also occasionally attacks can break through at other times.

Riding a bicycle or a horse are not infrequent causes of injury to children without any lapses of consciousness, though clearly the epileptic child is more at risk from developing injuries to both head and limb when falling. Of the two activities, cycling is the more dangerous, particularly because of the greater chance of problems arising with traffic. One should enquire as to what sort of cycling is envisaged. A child riding a tricycle around the garden is unlikely to suffer serious injury, whereas a teenager riding his cycle 5 miles to school through busy traffic would be at considerable risk, although it is not against the law. It is up to you to explain the problem to the family and for them to make the decision. On balance if a child is well controlled, the risks of just cycling away from traffic are not enormous and parents may decide to allow this. The problems with riding a horse are much less frequent and hazardous. The horse very often does the sensible thing, even when the rider is in a trance on his back. Clearly a serious injury might result from a child having a major tonic–clonic seizure while astride a horse and not being able to protect himself on falling off.

When an epileptic child goes swimming, he must be accompanied by someone specifically looking after him who is capable of rescuing him. He shouldn't just go as one of a crowd, because with the excitement in the pool, it is very easy for someone to be drowning when people think he is just swimming under water. The child shouldn't be allowed to go out of his own depth or, even more important, to go out of his minder's depth. He shouldn't be allowed to swim in the sea, except for splashing around in the shallows. It is worth emphasizing here that the child shouldn't be allowed deep baths at home and should be advised against turning on the tap when he is in the bath.

As far as PE is concerned, there is usually no problem with exercises on the ground; the difficulties arise when the child starts to climb. He should certainly be discouraged from climbing wall bars, ropes or climbing frames, otherwise a severe injury might result from falling onto a hard gymnasium floor. The child and parent should be strongly reassured that there should be no problem with the major sports. There is no difficulty with playing football, tennis, squash or running, indeed two first division footballers are under the first author's care with epilepsy.

In the present medicolegal climate, you may be judged culpable if you have not explained the possible risks to the child and his parents, even if they haven't asked you specifically about the potential problems.

Question 2. Fit or faint?

A GP is called to see a taxi driver of 28 who has collapsed while watching a football match on television. His wife says that he went funny and pale and passed out on the floor. He was unconscious for a minute or so. He didn't wet himself. There are no abnormal findings. Can it safely be assumed that this was a faint and he be allowed to go back to work the next day?

Absolutely not! By far the most likely cause for his lapse of consciousness, under these circumstances, was a fit. Otherwise normal, healthy males do not faint when they are sitting down.

If no convincing, alternative diagnosis can be made then the patient should not drive, even socially, for at least 12 months and it is possible that he might never drive professionally again.

He shouldn't be given the devastating news on first contact but he must be advised that he should not drive until his problems have been sorted out.

The history is most important. Previous episodes of loss of consciousness in childhood or youth should be sought. The patient should be asked if he has had any recent illness, particularly one with delirium or whether he has had a head injury at any time. Family history should also be gone into. The possibility of a cardiac problem should be considered.

Usually the patient will offer spontaneous information on whether he was feeling unwell at the time, with a stomach upset, for example. His passing a large melaena stool later in the day might put an entirely different complexion on things.

He should be asked what was the first thing he could remember after recovery from the lapse of consciousness. If he could remember nothing until he was upstairs in bed it was almost certainly a fit. Muscle aching after the attack would also be a strong pointer to a seizure. It would be sensible to speak to the wife separately, asking whether there was any rigidity or twitching during the period of unconsciousness and whether her husband was confused on regaining consciousness.

Almost invariably, on examining a patient like this, there is very little to find. A cardiac arrhythmia or murmur should be noted and, of course, any focal neurological signs.

He should be referred to the neurological department for investigation. He will almost certainly have an ECG and also an EEG. If the EEG is abnormal with epileptic changes then it makes the management of the patient's driving considerably easier. On the assumption that it was a fit, he should have a CT scan because of the small possibility of an intracranial lesion. If one draws a blank, or if there are cardiological pointers, 24-hour cardiac monitoring should be carried out. If cardiac arrhythmia is found, then a cardiac opinion and appropriate antiarrhythmic treatment is indicated.

With no evidence of an EEG abnormality and no evidence of any structural lesion, then an anticonvulsant is not indicated after a single attack. In many cases all that remains is what is termed an 'unexplained loss of consciousness'. There is nothing wrong with this description. By using it, the temptation to affix a more definitive label on poor evidence is resisted.

It is essential to achieve the upper hand in managing such patients and I strongly advise against saying 'I don't know what the cause of your attack was', but rather that 'You and your wife have not given us enough evidence on which to make a firm diagnosis. I am therefore not in a position to reassure you that it won't happen again' and to go on to say that he should notify the Driving Licence Authority. They will almost certainly say that he should remain off driving socially for a period of 12 months. There is approximately a 40–50% chance of further loss of consciousness and if it occurs, it usually does so in the first 12 months. He will not be allowed to regain his professional licence for several years, because the evidence is that the chance of an accident as a result of illness is very much greater in the professional driver. A taxi driver may well be at the wheel for 8 hours a day, 6 days a week. Statistically the chances of something going wrong during this period are much higher than for a housewife who drives for 20 minutes to do the shopping once a week.

Question 3.   It is petit mal?

The parents of a 5-year-old apparently normal child come to see you. They say there is a family history of petit mal epilepsy in the aunts, uncles and cousins. What should they look for in their own child?

Parents should be:

- Advised to look for lapses of concentration at home and poor progress at school and also to wonder about any unexplained falls or accidents which could have been due to a momentary lapse of awareness.
- Advised to look out for photosensitivity with odd jerking movements or lapses of concentration when the child is exposed to a flickering TV or light.
- Warned about the possibility of myoclonic jerks, particularly early in the morning.

If any of these signs occur, the parents should be advised to bring the child to the family doctor for referral to a neurologist who will, in turn, arrange an EEG.

The parents should be reassured that the child will most likely grow out of such attacks in adulthood. They should, however, be warned regarding restriction of activities such as those in Question 1.

Question 4.   'Just a febrile convulsion'

How should one manage a 2-year-old child who has a febrile convulsion lasting 3 minutes during an attack of tonsillitis? Would management be different if the convulsion lasted 20 minutes? Should this child be started on long-term anticonvulsants? 'It was just a febrile convulsion, Mrs. Smith.' Comment.

'Just a febrile convulsion.' Although in most cases there is no need for alarm, if appropriate steps are not taken, some patients might suffer brain damage and go on to develop temporal lobe epilepsy later in life.

1. If the child has recovered by the time you arrive, reduce pyrexia by removing clothing, tepid sponging and giving paracetamol. Then see the third point.
2. If the child is still convulsing, it would be ideal to give intravenous diazepam 0.15–0.25 mg/kg slowly over 5–10 minutes. Practically speaking, this is often very difficult and a satisfactory, much easier alternative is to give diazepam rectally – infinitely better than giving nothing at all. Give one 5 mg tube to infants aged 1–3 years. Over 3 years of age give a 10 mg tube. Do NOT give the diazepam by the intramuscular route as absorption is too slow and too unpredictable.
3. Decide on hospital admission when:
   • it is the first attack;
   • patient is under 18 months old;
   • there is a past history of series of attacks or prolonged attacks or focal component to present or past attack.

Definition: 'A febrile convulsion is a convulsion occurring with fever in a child aged 3 months to 5 years without any other obvious cause and without other evidence of epilepsy'.

Misunderstanding can arise. People with epilepsy are more likely to have a fit during a pyrexia than other times. So not all fits under the age of 5 years are febrile convulsions and epileptics can have a fit triggered by a pyrexia at any age.

Febrile convulsions are common. One child in 30 will have a single attack, one child in 100 will have two or more. Recurrent attacks are more likely when:

• There is a positive family history.
• The first convulsion occurred below the age of 15 months.
• The first convulsion was 15 minutes or longer.
• There were a series of attacks or focal features were present during attacks.

The history is very important. There may be a family history, not only of febrile convulsions, but also of epilepsy. Very often birth has not been perfectly normal – low birth weight, twins, breech, forceps delivery, prolonged or precipitate delivery. All might imply perinatal brain damage.

Recent head injury? Recent infection? Convulsions very often occur with the sudden rise in temperature at the start of an infection. How long did the fit last? Was there one or more? Were the twitches more on one side than the other suggesting unilateral focus?

Admission to hospital (see above) has the advantage that observation can be continued at night. If the child is kept at home one of the parents should stay up to ensure that no further convulsions have occurred and if they do occur, to take appropriate action.

Thirty per cent of children who have had a febrile convulsion will have further attacks, particularly if there is a family history or a history of birth trauma. Three per cent of the children will develop epilepsy in later life.

Febrile convulsions DO indicate a low convulsive threshold. Febrile convulsions CAN cause brain damage, particularly to the temporal lobe thereby providing a focus in a patient with a low epileptic threshold. This can, in turn, produce troublesome temporal lobe epilepsy later in life. For this reason, every effort must be made to truncate attacks.

A convulsion is an extremely frightening event for loving parents to witness in an infant. Those without previous experience will immediately assume that the child is going to die. The doctors faced with what, to him or her, is also a worrying situation must first reassure them and control their panic. If this isn't done, the parents will live in dread not only of further febrile convulsions in the child, but also of their own reaction to them.

'Rectal diazepam for the child, oral diazepam for the parents, and a whisky and water for the doctor.'

Antibiotics can be given in addition to paracetamol unless the infection is obviously viral, e.g. mumps. The argument that antibiotic treatment might conceal early meningitis can be countered by the fact that it might reduce the chance of a meningeal infection developing. The early use of antibiotics in a child prone to convulsions may prevent a further attack. The parents should certainly be instructed in using rectal diazepam and given a small supply of it to use at the first sign of trouble.

Should oral anticonvulsants be used in secondary prevention? I would favour trying the child on oral phenobarbitone for 12 months at least because it has been shown to reduce the recurrence rate by 50%. However, if there are any side effects, e.g. hyperactivity, then the phenobarbitone should be gradually withdrawn and stopped. Sodium valproate has also been shown to reduce the recurrence rate of febrile convulsions, but it is not marketed for such in the UK. There is no evidence that phenytoin or carbamazepine are of protective value in febrile convulsions although this may be a fault of the clinical trials rather than of the drugs themselves.

Certainly if there is any other evidence of epilepsy, for example fits occurring at times other than when the child is pyrexial, episodes of petit mal or absence attacks or an abnormal EEG, then prophylactic oral anticonvulsants should be tried. If there are focal features, then probably carbamazepine is the drug of choice. This treatment should be instituted by a paediatric or neurological specialist after careful assessment of the patient.

Immunization
Children with a history of febrile convulsions or those with a sibling who has had a febrile convulsion should be encouraged to receive immunization. There is unfortunately still a tendency to avoid immunizing such children. The only immunization which should be avoided in a child who has had a febrile convulsion is that against pertussis. A sibling of a child with febrile convulsions who has no other contra-indication can be safely immunized with pertussis vaccine. It should be explained to the parents that the risks of further febrile convulsions, if for example the child gets measles, are many times greater than if the child is vaccinated against measles.

Question 5. Temper or temporal lobe epilepsy?

A girl aged 16 has sudden outbursts of temper bordering on rage. She is aggressive and violent. When she settles down, she is remorseful and apologetic. What might indicate that these attacks are caused by temporal lobe epilepsy and not by an emotional or personality problem? What treatment would be available?

By far the most likely explanation for the attacks is that they are due to a behaviour disorder. However, the other two possibilities are that the girl is suffering from intermittent epileptiform discharges which produce the bursts of aggression or that she is disinhibited from some organic brain disorder.

A most useful question is: 'What appears to trigger the attacks?' If they have come on during non-appropriate times, or on occasions that have no manipulative value, or do not result from frustration or do not provide a defence against criticism – such as being told off for coming in late – then an organic lesion is more likely. Drug or solvent abuse must be borne in mind. Whatever the cause of the outbursts, they could be worse during menstruation and the premenstrual period.

Referral to a neurologist is indicated if there is any question of a temporary 'trance' or 'detachment' at the time of these attacks. EEG may help to clarify the matter. Carbamazepine is useful both in the treatment of temporal lobe epilepsy AND adolescent behavioural disturbance so its successful use might not throw much light on the diagnosis.

Question 6.   First fit at 53

A GP is called to see a railway worker of 53 who is a non-smoker and not a heavy drinker who has had a sudden tonic–clonic seizure. There is no previous history and no family history. He seems to be recovering quite well. What should influence the doctor to hospitalize him as an emergency? If he does not require admission, should a request be made for an urgent or a non-urgent outpatient appointment?

There is usually no need for urgent hospitalization after a single fit. However, if as a cause or as a result of it the patient has sustained a head injury, then he should be admitted for observation. Similarly if the patient strikes you as ill, especially if he is pyrexial with neck stiffness or if you are worried about the possibility of papilloedema, then he should be admitted promptly.

The causes for an isolated convulsion in a man of this age are shown in Table 1.

Table 1 Causes of isolated convulsion in an adult

Cerebral tumour – secondary or primary
Cerebral vascular disease
Cortical atrophy
Infection, meningitis, cerebral abscess or encephalitis
Drug induced, especially alcohol, antidepressants and phenothiazines
Head injury
Idiopathic

One should request an urgent outpatient appointment if the patient has been having headaches, especially if they have been suggestive of raised intracranial pressure, if there is any hint of any focal symptom or sign or if the relatives have noted any change in behaviour or intellectual performance.

I think ideally all patients who have had an isolated convulsion should have an early outpatient appointment and scan, because to most people it is a particularly unnerving experience and they feel that there must be something very seriously wrong to produce such an attack out of the blue. They will tend to be very dissatisifed with an appointment several months hence. Furthermore, having had a convulsion would probably have serious implications as far as driving and work are concerned.

Most patients should be advised before they go for their outpatient appointment that they should not drive (the Driving Licence Authority will usually request a 12-month period of observation before resuming driving, provided the EEG is normal). If you do not warn the patient at this stage and an accident happens as a result of a further lapse of consciousness, then you may be judged to be liable and action might be taken against you if any serious damage has been caused.

Normally anticonvulsants are not advised after a single attack, unless the EEG is frankly epileptic. Otherwise it would not be known whether the subsequent fit-free period was as a result of anticonvulsant therapy or not.

Question 7. First fit at 14

A boy of 14 has a sudden unexplained grand mal attack; there is a family history of epilepsy. He recovers completely. Should his doctor hospitalize him? If outpatient assessment is required, should an urgent or non-urgent appointment be requested?

I would only consider hospitalizing the boy if he has another fit on the same day or if he has clearly had a head injury or if he shows any signs of systemic illness, particularly fever. I would hospitalize him for observation if I felt the home circumstances were not satisfactory and he wouldn't be monitored properly at home.

The causes for fits at this age are shown in Table 2. In this particular boy's case, with a positive family history, it is very likely that he will have constitutional epilepsy and will not have an organic structural cause for his attack.

There is rarely any medical justification for requesting an urgent outpatient appointment for a patient of this nature, because a structural cause is so unlikely, but in view of the invariable parental concern, it is kind to see the patient as early as possible. If the boy has another fit before his outpatient appointment is due, then attempts should be made to bring the outpatient appointment forward so that treatment could be started as soon as possible after his second attack.

It is important to advise the patient and the family after an isolated convulsion that, for a period of observation, the boy should not cycle or climb, swim unattended or have deep baths. Otherwise if tragedy occurs, the doctor who has failed to give the appropriate warnings might be prosecuted.

Table 2 Causes of epilepsy in a 14-year-old boy

Constitutional/idiopathic epilepsy
Trauma
Infection
(Cerebral tumours at this age are almost always in the posterior fossa and therefore do not produce convulsions)

Question 8.   Alcohol withdrawal epilepsy

A man of 40 who drinks very heavily and has done for some years, suddenly decides to abstain completely. Four days after the last drink, he has a major convulsion. How would you regard this for the purposes of investigation, treatment, driving and working with machinery?

- It is safest to manage this patient in the same way as if he had presented with an isolated fit for which there was no immediately apparent cause.
- He should be told that he must stop driving at once.
- He should be told that it would be sensible not to work with dangerous machinery for the time being.
- He should be referred for full investigation and be told that his future management and treatment would depend on the results of such investigation.

Alcohol is a convulsant drug and, when taken acutely in excess, can produce tonic-clonic seizures. Conversely, when a moderate to heavy drinker suddenly stops drinking, he may suffer convulsions as a result of alcohol withdrawal. A fit occurring 4 days after withdrawal could still be alcohol related but other possibilities must be considered.

People who drink heavily are not immune to cerebral tumours, primary or secondary or vascular diseases and they are more prone than normal to cortical atrophy and to head injuries. Patients are sometimes prompted into stopping drinking because they feel unwell and it may be the combination of factors that has produced this fit.

Neurological referral is advisable in most cases. Every patient should have an ECG and some may require a 24-hour ECG monitoring, because occasionally a cardiac arrhythmia producing a sudden fall in cardiac output and cerebral perfusion will result in a tonic–clonic seizure. Chest X-ray to exclude a bronchial primary is essential and a full blood count may reveal a high mean corpuscular volume (MCV) and liver function tests and gamma GT may be abnormal. An EEG and CT scan should be performed in all such cases.

Usually after a single seizure, anticonvulsants are withheld unless there are very clear epileptic changes on the EEG. However, if the CT scan shows evidence of cerebral tumour, then anticonvulsants should be prescribed. Patients with normal EEGs and CT scans should perhaps be given multivitamins and they may require night sedation to prevent their drinking 'just to sleep'.

As far as driving is concerned, they would normally be allowed to resume driving their private cars after 12 months' freedom from further attacks. However the Driving Licence Authority will not consider them suitable for continuing to drive heavy goods vehicles or to have a public service vehicle licence. The latter includes taxis, private hire cars, ambulance, fire brigade and police driving.

Regulations as far as working with dangerous machinery are concerned are less clear cut. Some companies will not consider a patient working with dangerous machinery again if he has had a tonic–clonic seizure without warning, mainly because the insurance companies involved will not cover the individual concerned. If the patient is self-employed and willing to take risks, he should certainly be advised to avoid using exposed machinery for a period of 12 months, because if another attack is going to occur, the chances are that it will happen within this period. Often it is possible to find alternative employment in a big company, but in some instances this is not possible and some retraining may be necessary. To arrange this, he should contact the District Rehabilitation Officer.

Question 9.   Disco disaster – the flicker fit

A girl of 17 normally in perfect health has an epileptic attack during a prolonged sequence of stroboscopic lighting at a discotheque. Is this necessarily an event of prognostic significance? Can the same thing occur while watching television, in front of a computer screen or in any other circumstances?

- An epileptic attack, irrespective of the circumstances under which it occurred, is always of significance.
- Photosensitive convulsions can occur in many, varied situations.

The usual assumption under these circumstances is that the girl is photo-sensitive and has had a convulsion triggered by the flashing light. However, other things may have been, in part, responsible. It might, for example, be late at night, she has gone without sleep, there is often a higher level of excitement than usual and unfortunately she might have had too much alcohol.

Photosensitive convulsions also occur in young people when they approach a TV set to adjust it. The flickering on the screen when a child's eyes are very close to it is a particularly potent stimulus. This can happen when fiddling with the video recorder and trying to find the right place on the tape. Such incidents rarely occur with visual display units attached to professional computers, but are becoming more of a concern with the widespread use of computer games by children.

A particularly worrying situation is the likelihood of flicker-induced convulsion while driving. This happens typically with sunlight through a line of trees or railings, but it can also occur when driving through tunnels which are lit by strip lighting, for example on the M25.

There is often a family history and referral to a neurologist is advised.
An EEG will be required but a CT scan only rarely. Appropriate advice
regarding driving should be given (see Question 99). Photosensitivity
tends to decrease as patients enter their twenties.

Question 10.   The doctor, the Driving Licence Authority and the driver with epilepsy

**A 40-year-old sales executive comes to the surgery with a history of
at least two fits in the previous 3 months. An outpatient appointment
for him to see the neurologist is arranged. He is told that he must
notify the Driving Licence Authority and, above all, that he must not
drive. A week later, his GP sees him driving his company car down
the high street. Should the GP tell the Driving Licence Authority or
the man's company?**

Not immediately. No.

To tell the company or company doctor that the man does not comply
with the regulations and is driving against your advice constitutes a
breach of medical confidence and the patient might take action against
you even though he is clearly in the wrong.

It is essential, though, if you do see people in these circumstances that
you explain to them that they are not complying with the driving regulations and make it clear to them that you have recorded that warning in
your notes.

Very often the patients who are most insistent on their need to
continue driving are those who drive for a living or do so as part of their
job and these, of course, are the very people who are at greatest risk both
to themselves and to the public at large.

The patient may well protest that the attacks occurred under special
circumstances or suggest another factor which might be incorrect, but
appropriate, such as alcohol overindulgence. The Driving Licence
Authority tends to dismiss alcohol as an excuse for an attack because
patients who drink heavily and have lost consciousness are in a higher
risk group for further trouble.

Write to the patient, therefore, noting your observation, saying that
perhaps he misunderstood you. Confirm that he is not complying with
the driving regulations, that he should notify them and not drive again
until they say that he may resume. Point out that, whether he notifies
them or not, his insurance policy is now invalid. This very often does the
trick. You might also invite him to come along and discuss the matter
with you.

If the patient fails to heed your further warning, you should contact
your medical defence society and discuss with them what you should do.

Usually an acceptable approach is to write to the patient again and offer to write to the Driving Licence Authority on his behalf. The wording of the letter clearly needs to be tailored to the individual case and copies should be sent to the defence society. You may, however, decide that in the case of a bus driver, for example, your greater responsibility is to the public safety and feel that you must take some further action. Before you do, contact your defence society. For disclosure of medical information in public interest, without patient consent, see GMC publication *Professional Conduct and Discipline: fitness to practice.*

Question 11.   Shift work – more fits?

A factory worker of 28 finds that his mortgage repayments are causing him a lot of anxiety. He intends to change to shift work. However he has occasional tonic–clonic epilepsy and is on pheno-barbitone and phenytoin for this. Is it likely that his fits will get worse? How should he be advised?

The fits may well become more frequent.

The main worry is that the change in sleep pattern, which usually means reduction in sleep, will cause an exacerbation of his epilepsy. Shift work usually means spending some days or weeks working mornings, afternoons and then nights. This is much more disruptive than someone who goes on to permanent night work.

The history may be very helpful. If he has had fits in the past that were clearly related to loss of sleep, then he would be well advised not to take up shift work, but to think of an alternative way of improving his income.

The point of changing to shift work is obviously a good occasion for checking the patient's anticonvulsant medication; it might be worth checking his anticonvulsant level and advising an increase in medication if the levels are surprisingly low. One should also give him advice about ensuring that the change in lifestyle does not mean that he would be forgetting to take some of his pills and a new pattern would have to be constructed.

It is worth checking that while a man is taking on his new position because it is more lucrative, it does not involve change in work such that he is going to work on dangerous or exposed machinery. The risks involved here may be judged to be unacceptable.

It is also worth checking on how he is going to get to and from work. It is possible that he has been driving against advice and hasn't thought of getting to work at unsociable hours by any other means. If he has gone for 1 year without an attack, then one would hope that he would not have a fit as a result of changing his lifestyle, because if he did it would mean that he wouldn't be able to drive for a period of 1 year and this might make transport to and from work impossible.

Question 12. 'If I leave her she might suffocate'

A man works shifts and one week in four is away all night. His wife has started to suffer from occasional nocturnal fits and he is afraid that left alone she might suffocate. What advice would you give?

I would advise that:

- The patient should be allowed just one foam pillow rather than large feather-filled ones.
- Hard sharp-edged bedside furniture should be removed.
- The bed should not be high off the ground and the floor should be thickly carpeted so that the chances of significant injury are minimized in the event of the patient projecting herself out of bed.
- False teeth and plates should be removed.
- If the patient tends to vomit during convulsions she should avoid having food for at least 3 hours before she goes to bed.
- To prevent the patient lying awake for hours worrying about the security in her husband's absence, effort should be made to convince her that the house is safe from intruders.

There is common concern among the loved ones of epileptics that, left alone, they might suffer some serious bodily harm. Parents are particularly anxious about the risk to their children when they move away from home to live alone, to go to college or university for example. Some people do, in fact, suffer awful injuries, burns, etc. during a fit and occasionally they can be found dead. When this occurs during the night, the explanations are that the patient has gone into an attack of status epilepticus from which she didn't recover, that the patient aspirated vomit and suffocated or that a head injury was sustained. But for all this, such occurrences are rare.

Question 13. Epilepsy and oral contraceptives

What advice should be given to a girl of 18 who suffers from epilepsy and who wishes to go on to the oral contraceptive?

She can be told that 'the Pill' is unlikely to upset her epilepsy. Indeed, some girls find that their epilepsy improves when they start to take oral contraceptives. There is one problem, however. Because of the enzyme induction caused by anticonvulsants, particularly phenytoin and carbamazepine, she should be advised to take a pill containing at least 50 µg of oestrogen. She should also be even more careful than usual about not missing a pill. If particularly anxious about avoiding pregnancy a condom could be used in mid-cycle.

Question 14. Prescribing in pregnancy

A woman of 27 who suffers from moderately well controlled tonic–clonic seizures intends to start a family. She is worried that her medication might cause a fetal abnormality. What would you say to her? Might you change her treatment?

- I would reassure her that, generally, there is little risk of teratogenicity, less than from the epilepsy not being well controlled.
- I would take the opportunity of assessing her anticonvulsant therapy and make any necessary changes.

There is some slight increased risk of teratogenicity in epileptics, possibly as a result of some genetic factors and also from the effect of having major convulsions. Minor convulsions probably have no significant impact. Added to this, there is concern that some anticonvulsants may be teratogenic and obviously it is towards these that the patient's attention is directed. It is very important to put this into perspective and to tell patients how silly it is to worry about anticonvulsants if they continue to smoke or drink alcohol.

It should also be emphasized that the benefits gained from preventing many major fits are more valuable than the potentially harmful effects of some of the drugs.

The young couple coming for advice about anticonvulsant therapy before embarking on pregnancy present one with a golden moment for reconsideration of the patient's management and for attempting to improve therapy with the full cooperation of the family.

First, is she on appropriate therapy? A change may be required. She may still be on ethosuximide and no longer at risk from petit mal attacks. She may be on valproate for what is essentially a focal epilepsy with generalized spread. For generalized seizures in the adult with a hemisphere focus, carbamazepine is the drug of choice. It is probable that multiple anticonvulsant therapy exposes the patient to greater risk than monotherapy which is guided by blood anticonvulsant levels. So one would advise a gradual change to monotherapy with, say, carbamazepine. Sodium valproate should be slowly withdrawn if possible because of the slight risk of neural tube defects. The anticonvulsant removed must be reduced very slowly, e.g. with phenytoin 50 mg per fortnight and with valproate 200 mg per fortnight. The blood level of the remaining drug should be kept in the lower half of the recommended range, provided this is adequate to suppress attacks. It is important to advise any change in therapy BEFORE the woman becomes pregnant. Once pregnant, the most sensible advice is to avoid sudden changes in antiepileptic drugs because if such changes are made, major convulsions might ensue with possibly damaging effect.

If a woman is happy on valproate or phenytoin, the advice is that she continues on it, with a check being made on her blood anticonvulsant levels. If she is on phenytoin and is only moderately well controlled and has never tried carbamazepine, then it might be sensible to attempt to switch her to carbamazepine protection. When carbamazepine is being introduced, it should be increased very slowly by, say, just 50 mg every 4–5 days. It should also be emphasized that a reasonable level of carbamazepine should be achieved before the pre-existing anticonvulsant is reduced.

However, if starting the family is imminent, then the best advice would be to maintain her on phenytoin because of the risk of convulsions being higher during the period of change-over. Again, the blood levels should be checked to make sure they are in the lower half of the recommended therapeutic range.

There is a temptation to try withdrawal of phenobarbitone or primidone. In the author's (DJT) experience, this has to be done extremely slowly because people who have been on these drugs for a long time tend to have considerable trouble with withdrawal convulsions.

It is important to warn the patient and the family that any reduction or change in anticonvulsant therapy may lead to an increase in the chance of convulsion. If a woman is only moderately well controlled, then clearly she would not comply with the driving regulations. If the patient is driving, then it must be emphasized that she would have to stop driving while the changes are being achieved and for a period of observation on the new therapy. Many patients find stopping driving unacceptable and decide to remain on their previous medication.

Once the first 12 weeks of pregnancy have passed, the risk of teratogenicity ceases. Phenytoin, however, is thought to produce growth retardation in some cases. It is important to appreciate that the need for anticonvulsant drugs often goes up in the last third of the pregnancy and the dose needs to be increased – again check blood levels. Maternal serum α-fetoprotein, ultrasound and, in selected cases, amniocentesis are to be recommended to detect signs of fetal abnormality in early pregnancy. Remember to give folic acid supplements.

Question 15. Aiming for the safe delivery

A rather small woman with constitutional epilepsy is pregnant. Would it be a good idea for her to have an elective caesarean section?

Yes. Most probably.

The tendency for epilepsy and a low convulsive threshold to be inherited has been estimated at approximately 1 in 6. If one adds to this a significant perinatal head injury and anoxia, then a new neurological patient is born.

Nowadays, epileptic women should be very carefully assessed. By using ultrasound measurements, one should be able to tell pelvic size and fetal head size accurately and obviously one can have a clear picture of presentation. Babies that are likely to be born by breech presentation and twin pregnancies should probably be delivered by caesarean section.

If a perfectly normal vaginal delivery is to be expected without there being any delay in labour or the need for instruments, then a normal vaginal delivery can be recommended. However, if there is any question of doubt, and doubt can have a broad spectrum, then a caesarean section should be discussed with the patient and her husband.

If the woman or her husband raised the question of whether she should have a caesarean section, then it is a very brave obstetrician or GP who advises against it without having shown very careful consideration and assessment of the problem in general. It is important that a joint decision is reached and that the patient has been fully informed of the slightly increased risk to herself that caesarean section entails.

Question 16. Anticonvulsants and anticoagulants

A man of 50 who suffers from epilepsy develops a deep vein thrombosis. What problems can arise when a person on anticonvulsants also has to take anticoagulants?

The two main problems which can arise are:

- The effects of injury.
- Interaction between the two types of drug.

The main concern is that if a patient has a major tonic–clonic seizure while on anticoagulants, he may injure his head and produce a serious intracranial haemorrhage, possibly fatal. Obviously other injuries can occur with much more bleeding than usual, but hopefully without fatal consequences.

A secondary concern is that there are drug interactions between anticonvulsants and anticoagulants which make anticoagulation somewhat less predictable. The usual situation here is that a patient is already on anticonvulsants and then needs to be anticoagulated. A patient might, for example, be on anticonvulsants following a craniotomy or head injury and then develop a deep vein thrombosis or pulmonary embolism. A similar situation arises when people with convulsions and vascular disease need to be put on anticoagulants because their transient ischaemic attacks fail to respond to aspirin and dipyridamole.

Providing patients are maintained on the same dose of anticonvulsant, no great difficulty should be encountered in achieving a reliable anticoagulant level. The dose of anticoagulant, however, will be quite different from that needed in a similar patient not on anticonvulsants.

Occasionally a patient who is on anticoagulants, for one reason or another starts to have fits and requires anticonvulsant therapy. When an anticonvulsant has to be introduced in these circumstances, the dose of the anticoagulant will almost invariably need to be changed and usually the dose needs to be increased – there is a complex interaction between protein binding and enzyme induction. The safest thing is to do the prothrombin time frequently and adjust the anticoagulant dose accordingly.

Clearly the combination of anticonvulsants and anticoagulants is to be avoided whenever possible. If it is unavoidable, then the counsel of perfection is to keep the patient on anticoagulants for as short a time as possible.

Question 17.   Depression and epilepsy

A woman of 45 has a long history of tonic–clonic seizures which are well controlled on phenobarbitone and phenytoin. She develops a fairly severe endogenous depression. How should one proceed?

- Check blood levels of anticonvulsant(s).
- Consider changing anticonvulsant medication, particularly with regard to phenobarbitone.
- If severe depression exists and antidepressants HAVE to be used, bear in mind that tricyclics and tetracyclics are potentially epileptogenic; low dose flupenthixol (0.5 to 1.0 mg) twice daily may be tried.
- ECT must not be used in epileptics.

This is a common problem and an important question which has several facets and many different courses of action. The commonly used antidepressants, for example the tricyclics and tetracyclics, have convulsant properties and all the anticonvulsants can produce endogenous depression. In this particular case, the patient might have depression as a result of anticonvulsant therapy or she might be depressed because she has been denied having convulsions or it may just be coincidental.

It has been observed that allowing a depressed patient to have a convulsion might improve that patient's mood but, with all the implications regarding injury, work and driving, this is not recommended.

The anticonvulsants most likely to contribute towards depression are phenobarbitone and primidone. The least likely to cause trouble of this kind are carbamazepine and lamotrigine.

The first thing to check, therefore, is the patient's blood level and if either anticonvulsant is producing unacceptably high levels; simply reducing the dose to bring the level into the recommended therapeutic range may be enough to improve the patient's mood. If the drug levels are satisfactory, then it would be sensible to consider reducing and eventually stopping the phenobarbitone, if the patient is willing to accept the possibility of having a withdrawal convulsion. If the depression continues when the patient is on phenytoin alone, then consider gradually changing her over to carbamazepine, substituting approximately 100 mg carbamazepine for every 50 mg phenytoin per week. Lamotrigine would be a satisfactory alternative. The patient must be reminded again that a withdrawal convulsion is possible and for this reason, she should be advised against driving, if she previously satisfied the driving regulations. She should be advised against driving if an antidepressant with convulsant properties is prescribed.

As far as specific treatment for the depression is concerned, the patient should certainly not have ECT. In the epileptic, ECT can sometimes cause a fatal status epilepticus.

Low dose flupenthixol is currently the antidepressant of choice in epileptics. Fluoxetine and paroxetine may also be considered as the associated risk of increasing fits is likely to be small.

Question 18.   Phenytoin – getting the right level

Mrs Black's epilepsy is well controlled on her dose of phenytoin. A blood test shows the anticonvulsant level to be below the recommended therapeutic range. Mrs White's epilepsy is not well controlled by her dose of phenytoin, although her blood test shows the anticonvulsant level is well within the therapeutic range. How would you advise these women?

- I would tell Mrs Black to stay on the same dose.
- In Mrs White's case either her epilepsy would never be satisfactorily controlled by anticonvulsants or phenytoin might not be the right drug for her. I would assume the latter and would change her to another anticonvulsant.

Some patients seem controlled by a dose of phenytoin which gives a blood level less than that recommended. It could be argued, in such a case as Mrs Black, that the phenytoin might no longer be needed at all and could be discontinued. The largest problem arising from this is that the patient would have to stop driving for an observation period (possibly 6 months) to make sure she didn't have a phenytoin withdrawal convulsion. If the phenytoin level is surprisingly low, it is always as well to check that the patient took the last dose before the blood test. Sometimes patients will forget to do so and also neglect to tell you that they had forgotten.

In Mrs White's case, however, is she on the appropriate anticonvulsant for her type of epilepsy? If it was myoclonic epilepsy, for example, she would be better off on a benzodiazepine such as nitrazepam. For photosensitive attacks, sodium valproate would be the drug of choice and for petit mal, had it continued into adulthood, sodium valproate or ethosuximide.

For most other types of epilepsy, the three drugs other than phenytoin that could be considered would be carbamazepine, primidone and sodium valproate. It would be worth transferring Mrs White from phenytoin to carbamazepine, but it would have to be pointed out to her that she might experience more fits during the time of transfer because the withdrawal of even an inadequate anticonvulsant can increase the number of attacks and, if done suddenly, can result in a possibly fatal status epilepticus.

Initially, the phenytoin dosage should be kept the same and carbamazepine introduced gradually, say 50 mg a day for a week, then increasing to 50 mg twice daily and so on until the patient is on 400 mg a day. The anticonvulsant levels could then be checked and, if satisfactory, the patient kept on the old dose of phenytoin and the 400 mg carbamazepine a day and observed over a period to see whether the combination is more effective than phenytoin. If it is, then the phenytoin could be gradually reduced and the carbamazepine levels checked, initially every month (because of drug interaction between phenytoin and carbamazepine) and the daily dose of carbamazepine adjusted according to the blood level and also to the patient's symptoms if she develops any side effects. In some instances the patient will be satisfactorily controlled on the carbamazepine, but in others it may be necessary to reintroduce phenytoin, keeping her on two anticonvulsants (provided the combination was shown to be of more benefit than either drug alone). Alternatively, one could gradually switch her over from carbamazepine to primidone or sodium valproate.

It must be emphasized that it is not in the patient's interests to change anticonvulsants frequently or quickly. Epilepsy is a cyclical disorder and when the patient is going through a difficult phase is not a good time to consider modifying therapy, beyond checking blood levels and increasing as necessary. It should be explained to the epileptic that if she were on no anticonvulsant at all, she would have trouble-free phases and then a bad cluster when vulnerable.

Question 19.   Flying and epilepsy

Are there any circumstances in which a person with a past history of epilepsy, now well controlled, may hold a private pilot's licence?

No. But there is no objection to a well-controlled epileptic flying as a passenger.

People who are flying should be reminded to:

- Pack their anticonvulsants and take them regularly.
- Avoid alcohol on the flight.
- Avoid sleep-depriving night flights if possible.

Headaches

Question 20. What is a significant headache?

A man of 38 has had a headache for 3 weeks. What factors would make you feel that the headaches were of pathological significance? How long do you think the headaches should be allowed to continue without a neurological opinion?

The following factors would make me suspect that the headaches were of pathological significance:

● Present on waking.
● The headache increases with manoeuvres raising intracranial pressure, for example coughing, sneezing and straining.
● If there are any associated neurological symptoms.
● If there are any associated neurological signs.
● If the characteristics of the headache did not suggest migraine or muscular contraction headache (tension headache).

If you suspect raised intracranial pressure – phone for an appointment.

Present on waking
The headache of raised intracranial pressure is typically worse when the patient first wakes up and then begins to subside as he gets up and around. Lying flat all night has a gravitational effect on increasing cerebral oedema. This type of headache should be distinguished from the headache of depression where the patient will often wake without headache but it comes on while he is still in bed and then it may increase in severity when he attempts to become involved in the day. The early morning headache of cervical spondylosis is unlikely to be found in a 38 year old.

Muscular contraction headaches typically come on in the late afternoon and early evening, but they can be present first thing in the morning, particularly if the patient has had a restless night with bad dreams and periods of semi-consciousness where there has been wrestling with unresolved worries.

Migrainous neuralgia may wake patients in the middle of the night and often you will have a story of someone being woken between 2 and 3 a.m. every night of the week. These headaches can also occur at a sterotyped time during the day. There is often history of a previous cluster and the head pain is accompanied by a ptosis, watering of the eye and blockage of the nose on the painful side.

Aggravating features
One should always ask what makes the headache better or worse. With

cerebral tumour, the head pain is likely to increase when the patient strains at stool or coughs or sneezes, although these changes may also occur in muscular contraction headache or migraine. Patients with cerebral tumour are not usually photophobic and surprisingly their headache is relieved by simple analgesics, at least initially, while many patients with muscular contraction headache have no such relief.

Associated neurological symptoms

Patients with cerebral tumour may have vomiting with little or no preceding nausea. However, many such patients are troubled by nausea and one may be misled into believing that they have migraine. Analgesics taken for the headache may well produce nausea and vomiting in the susceptible.

One should ask for the symptoms of diplopia or any hemi-phenomenon with unilateral difficulties with manipulation or changes in sensation and one should also enquire after changes in mood, motivation and attacks of disturbed consciousness.

Associated neurological signs

Papilloedema – there is quite rightly an obsession with looking for papilloedema and, when it is found, it clearly puts a whole new complexion on the clinical problem. However, it should be emphasized that some patients never develop papilloedema, however high their intracranial pressure rises. On the other hand, long-sighted individuals usually have small, slightly red discs which are sometimes wrongly diagnosed as papilloedematous.

It is always worth looking quickly for a visual field defect because, surprisingly, field defects of gradual onset are often overlooked by the patient. Abnormal eye movements, especially when accompanied by diplopia of recent onset, are also important. Difficulties in interpretation may arise in patients with longstanding squint. Look for minor degrees of imbalance and evidence of minor clumsiness or weakness on either side and test for any difference in sensation between the two sides. Obviously, any difference in the reflexes should be taken very seriously.

Atypical headache

One should always be particularly cautious about patients whose description of the headache does not comply with muscular contraction headache or any of the varieties of migraine i.e.

1. Common migraine – usually a unilateral headache ± anorexia, ± nausea, with occasional vomiting.
2. Classical migraine – as 'common migraine' with visual symptoms.
3. Hemiplegic, or focal, migraine – as above with hemi-phenomena, i.e. dysphasia, hemiparesis or hemi-anaesthesia.

4. Complicated migraine – where neurological signs persist after acute attack (most commonly, homonymous hemianopia).
5. Migrainous neuralgia (syn. 'cluster headaches') – severe periorbital pain, ± red eye, ± watering of eye, ± nasal blockage, every day at approximately the same time.

Muscular contraction, or 'tension', headache also has very specific features: occurring virtually every day, for most of the day, although tending to be worse in the afternoon and evening, described as a tight band around the head or a bursting sensation or a pressure or weight on the top of the head and associated with a tightness in the muscles at the back of the neck. Often the pain is severe and the patient will have little relief from analgesics. If the nature of the headache is obscure, then it is important to keep the patient under observation and possibly to refer, if improvement fails to occur.

Timing of neurological referral
Clearly the patient should be referred promptly if there are any of the worrying features present which have been mentioned above. Don't just send a routine letter to outpatient appointments – phone up.

All patients with recent onset of headache, or those in whom there has been a recent change in the character of their headache, should be kept under regular review. If they fail to improve after 2–3 weeks, they should be referred on for a neurological consultation.

Question 21.　Do brain tumours run in the family?

A man aged 47 complains of a headache. He says that 3 months ago his brother died of a brain tumour. Should one take his headache more seriously, less seriously or with equal seriousness in comparison with any other patient?

- The patient will need to be taken more seriously. Certainly he will need more reassurance than the average.
- It would be wise to enquire after the nature of the brother's tumour.

The lesion may have been a secondary deposit which would make the situation commonplace. Some rare primary tumours do have a family history. Some families seem to be particularly prone to cancer. There are accounts of families with several gliomas in their pedigree. In any event, in a case like this, I would advise erring on the side of caution and referring if at all concerned.

Question 22.   Early morning headache

A young female school-teacher wakes up every morning at 6.0 a.m. with an almost unbearable headache. Occasionally she vomits. She was investigated for headaches 3 months before and nothing was found. She was told that they were caused by stress. What should the GP do?

Re-refer to the neurologist! (This is important both for the patient and for the neurologist!)

You may well find that the character of the headache has changed since the patient was last assessed, making the diagnosis clearer. Although there are several causes of early morning headache (see Questions 20 and 70), one should always assume that early morning headaches in young people are due to raised intracranial pressure. She might have developed associated features, such as unilateral motor or sensory disturbances or balance or visual problems. When a patient first develops symptoms, she might not have papilloedema. At 3 months it would be much easier to detect.

The doctor should determine what her previous assessment and investigations included. Unfortunately, in many parts of the country with long neurological waiting lists, the patients are often seen by a non-neurologist and sometimes by a relatively inexperienced registrar. The investigations sometimes include just a blood count and a lateral skull X-ray and it must be ensured that a brain scan has been performed. However, even if it has been performed, it may be necessary to repeat it, because an X-ray CT brain scan may miss early tumours, particularly in the posterior fossa. Depending on the clinical features, the patient may be advised to have an MRI (magnetic resonance imaging) scan.

If no structural lesion is detected, then it may be necessary to perform a lumbar puncture and CSF pressure measurement. Raised pressure might be due to benign intracranial hypertension. This can be treated with acetazolamide or repeated lumbar punctures until spontaneous recovery occurs.

If the CSF pressure is within the normal range, then other causes for early morning headache would have to be reconsidered, such as depression, alcohol abuse or a cervical musculoskeletal problem. The latter often manifests itself in the morning because patients often tolerate, while asleep, distorted neck positions which they would not tolerate while awake.

Question 23.   The Earth moved! – coital migraine

A man of 43 develops a severe headache at orgasm. The pain takes about 10–15 minutes to subside and the man doesn't vomit. What is

the most likely diagnosis? What investigations should be undertaken, if any, and what advice should be given regarding further
intercourse?

- The most likely cause is coital migraine.
- The possibility of subarachnoid leak cannot be ignored. The patient
  should be referred for a neurological opinion and investigation as
  necessary.
- Various methods can be tried to prevent coital migraine.

A very sudden severe headache at the point of orgasm is not an
uncommon symptom and does not usually have a structural cause, but it
must be remembered that a subarachnoid bleed can occur at the moment
of orgasm and if there is any doubt an early referral should be made.
Lumbar puncture must be carried out within 2 weeks of the episode to
have any chance of being positive. In this particular patient the very
rapid resolution of the symptoms strongly suggests coital migraine.

If the diagnosis of coital migraine is made, the neurologist will give
reassurance and advice on dietary habits and physical and mental stress.
Occasionally, anti-migraine medication such as low dose clonidine,
pizotifen, even ergotamine, might be used in a prophylactic fashion.
Prolonged medication is unnecessary because the condition is self-
limiting.

Question 24.   Migraine and the Pill

A woman of 23 has increasingly severe migraine. She smokes and
takes oral contraceptives. She says that it is socially unacceptable for
her to become pregnant, and she will not contemplate any other
form of contraception. Is she at any risk? How would you advise?

Yes, she is at risk. She may have a stroke if she stays on the oral contraceptive pill, especially if she continues to smoke. I would advise her to
stop cigarettes and take one aspirin a day.

It is very common for migraine to be more frequent and more severe
on the oral contraceptive pill. Indeed some women only have migraine
when they are on the Pill. Paradoxically, a few (the lucky ones) have
fewer headaches when on the Pill. The real concern develops when a
patient has a dysphasia or a hemiparesis or hemi-anaesthesia. If these
focal symptoms occur, then most women do not need much persuading
to change their form of contraception.

Cerebral complications are much more likely to occur on high dose
oestrogen pills and in women who have been pregnant, even if the pregnancy was terminated.

If the migraine is worse on the contraceptive pill, provided there are no severe focal symptoms, the risks of stroke are small; you should attempt to transfer her to a progesterone-only pill or from a 50 µg oestrogen pill to one of the low dose 30 µg oestrogen pills. You should certainly stop the woman smoking and quite a sensible approach is to add a small dose of aspirin, say one enteric-coated aspirin per day. Not only will this have a useful antiplatelet action, but aspirin is quite an efficient migraine prophylactic. I would encourage her to take fish oil in the form of halibut liver oil capsules which may reduce the chances of unwanted thrombosis. If these simple measures are not enough to control the migraine, then ensure that she is not going without sleep or food and try adding another migraine prophylactic such as clonidine, pizotifen or a β-blocker. For the acute attacks use an anti-emetic with a simple soluble analgesic or sumatriptan. This $5HT_1$ agonist can be given by mouth or by self-injection – particularly useful if the patient is vomiting.

In conclusion, women whose migraine is worse on the oral contraceptive pill, especially if there are focal features, should be advised to stop, at least temporarily. If, as in the present case, advice to stop the oral contraceptive pill is unacceptable, taking these various precautions is probably safer than running the gauntlet of an unwanted pregnancy. For propaganda reasons, the severe cerebral vascular problems which can occur in pregnancy do not reach the front page of the tabloid press.

Question 25. Problem headaches

Some people seem to have their lives ruled by migraine, some have only occasional, but devastating, attacks and some people have common migraine mixed with muscular-contraction (tension) headaches. How would you manage:

1. **A patient on migraine prophylaxis who gets breakthrough attacks?**
2. **A businessman of 32 who has a severe migraine attack 3 or 4 times a year, often coinciding with an important business meeting?**
3. **A patient who has a probable combination of migraine and muscular-contraction headaches?**
4. **A patient who has cluster headaches (migrainous neuralgia)?**

1. You should think of attempting to improve the overall management of the patient by scrutinizing the diet. Note that apart from asking about dietary trigger factors, an important dietary factor may be going without food. You should try to ensure that the patient has enough but not too much sleep, to attempt to improve the life-style and the patient's understanding of trigger factors and to ensure that the

patient is on an appropriate dose of one of the two standard prophy-
lactics – pizotifen or propranolol. It might be worth switching to one
that has not previously been tried. The addition of half a soluble
aspirin a day to the prophylactic drug or taken alone can, in my
opinion, sometimes help. It may be necessary to stop the oral contraceptive pill or HRT.

For the almost inevitable breakthrough attack, many will obtain
relief by taking an analgesic like paracetamol or aspirin. It may be
worth adding an anti-emetic such as metoclopramide or domperidone. Even if the patient does not have prominent nausea and
vomiting there is often gastric stasis which these drugs may improve.
Giving the anti-emetic by a non-oral route can be of benefit. The
secret is to take the analgesic at the very first sign of a migraine
coming on and not to wait until the headache itself begins. Patients
who are good observers can often sense that they are in the prodromal
phase of a migraine when they might feel unaccountably tired or their
perceptions might be heightened or they develop a craving for certain
foods or drink – chocolate or coffee, for example!

Do not resort to opiates! If simple analgesics fail, go on to a
specific anti-migraine preparation such as sumatriptan.

Sumatriptan is a very effective drug but it cannot be used on everybody. It is contraindicated, for example, not just in patients with
known ischaemic heart disease but also in those in whom unrecog-
nized cardiac disease is a possibility without a prior evaluation of
such disease, e.g. post-menopausal women, males over 40 years and
patients with a risk factor of IHD. This is not necessarily as restrictive
as it sounds as a high proportion of severe migraine sufferers are in a
younger age group. There is no doubt that some people find that their
lives have been transformed by sumatriptan.

Use 50 mg by mouth or 6 mg by sub-cutaneous injection (a useful
route if the patient is nauseated or if particularly rapid relief is
required). In very many patients a dose of 50 mg is effective and may
be particularly appropriate if adverse effects or hepatic impairment
limit the use of the 100 mg tablets.

Sumatriptan should not be used if the patient has had ergotamine or
its derivatives within the last 24 hours or if the patient is on lithium or
on a selective 5HT re-uptake inhibitor or on an MAOI. After a good
response to the first dose the patient's symptoms may recur. If they
do, another tablet, or injection, can be tried (no more than 300 mg
tablets to be used within 24 hours and no more than 2 injections
within 24 hours).

A minority of sufferers may favour an ergotamine preparation (to
which the same restrictions, regarding ischaemic heart disease as
above, also apply). It is better to give ergotamine via a nasal spray,
sub-lingually or rectally, because it is not well absorbed orally.
Remember that it has a long half-life and if people take more than

8 mg a week they can develop ergotamine-induced headaches which are troublesome (see Question 27).

2. With a long interval between attacks, long-term prophylaxis is not indicated (only consider if the patient is having at least 3 migraine attacks per month). However, experience suggests that it may be helpful for the patient to take 10 mg of propranolol before a stressful event, provided of course that there is no history of asthma. The drug should first be practised with on one or two occasions at the weekend to make sure it does not have a bad effect on performance.

This man seems ideal for sumatriptan subcutaneous injection. Very often just having it with him in the briefcase will give that extra confidence, knowing that even though he has an attack, he can quickly do something about it.

3. This is a very common combination, particularly in teenagers in whom, for developmental reasons, a migraine and muscular-contraction headache frequently co-exist. The approach here is either to treat the migraine with a prophylactic or to treat the individual migrainous episodes efficiently depending upon their frequency. When this is done, the muscular-contraction headaches often subside.

In older patients, it is common to find the muscular-contraction headache element uppermost with the migraine being occasional. In this situation it is usually better, therefore, to direct the thrust of treatment towards the muscular-contraction headaches by trying to discover what has produced them. Very often it is a mild depression. This can make it difficult for the patient to cope with day-to-day activities as efficiently as previously and headaches will result. It is this group in which experience suggests that a low dose of an anti-depressant such as amitriptyline (10 mg at night) can be effective. Physiotherapy can also help to teach patients to relax the muscles of the neck and scalp. Sometimes the muscular-contraction headache has spread from stiffness in the neck and back caused by cervical spondylosis. In this group, a collar may be helpful.

4. A patient with cluster headaches does not normally require a prophylactic in between the clusters. However, during the vulnerable phase, the patient's head pains tend to occur at a predictable time, often waking him from sleep in the early hours of the morning. The old advice, in this situation, was to have a dose of ergotamine on retiring. Most patients, however, find sumatriptan very effective. A subcutaneous injection of sumatriptan given at the very first sign of an attack developing can give very considerable relief from this agonizing pain. Some patients also respond well to oxygen inhalation and can be provided with a cylinder and face mask for use at home. Oxygen works, in this context, as a cerebral vasoconstrictor.

Steroid treatment may also be tried during the few weeks of the

cluster. Often quite a high initial dose is required, i.e. 40 mg of prednisolone daily, with an attempt to reduce the dose by 5 mg per week.
Propranolol and clonidine do not seem to be very effective as prophy-
lactics during the vulnerable period, but pizotifen can be in a minority
of cases. Previously lithium was used in some patients but this is no
longer often the case as it denies patients the considerable benefits of
sumatriptan.

Question 26.   Hard work headache

**A boy is studying for his 'A' levels; every time he does more than a
little work involving concentration, he develops a 'migraine'. Should
he be advised to look for something other than an academic career?
Would it be worth using a β-blocker, a tranquillizer or some alternative type of medicine such as acupuncture or hypnosis?**

- This is unlikely to be simply migraine.
- It is necessary to make a clear diagnosis.
- Treatment is likely to be effective.
- There is usually no need to abandon an academic career but it may be
  necessary to reorientate it.

Headaches which occur every day are very unlikely to be migraine, the
only exception to this being migrainous neuralgia which would be
exceptional at this age. A much more likely explanation for the boy's
headaches is that he is having muscular-contraction headaches for most
of the time. Another possibility is that he is having so-called 'mixed
headaches', i.e. the occasional migraine headache perhaps once a week
or once a fortnight which sets the mould for a headache and, in between,
he is having muscular-contraction headaches.

It is essential to make a clear diagnosis. There could be pathological
causes, e.g. sinusitis, head injury, virus infection, depression, or
emotional causes, such as wrong 'A' level subjects, girl friend trouble,
family problems.

Certainly, treatment is indicated before a career is abandoned.
Hynotherapy is good for relaxation and self-hypnosis is sometimes
useful but acupuncture in this context is not often effective. Sometimes
this kind of headache will improve with a small dose of amitripyline
for 4–6 weeks (10 mg at night). If the boy is having migraine, in the
absence of asthma, a β-blocker would be an appropriate first choice
prophylactic or, failing that, pizotifen or low dose clonidine can be
tried. Acute attacks should be treated promptly with a combination of
an anti-emetic with an analgesic or the more specific anti-migraine
agent sumatriptan (however, sumatriptan is not licensed for children
under 18 years).

Question 27. Only ergot helps

A pre-menopausal woman of 48 has attacks of quite severe migraine. The only treatment that seems to help is ergotamine. During her premigrainous aura, she has tingling of the right side of her face and right hand. How would you deal with the case? Is ergotamine more dangerous in migraine with focal symptoms?

- A careful assessment should be made to confirm the diagnosis of migraine.
- If the diagnosis of migraine is established and no other risk factors are present, she should continue to use ergotamine in acute attacks. Other medication might be tried in addition.
- In spite of her focal signs, there is no conclusive evidence that ergotamine will make things worse. It is unlikely to increase the cerebral ischaemia.

This question raises several important issues. First, are the right-sided sensory attacks just migraine or are they transient cerebral ischaemic attacks due to thromboembolism, or are they possibly focal minor elipeptic attacks? In view of her age, is there likely to be a hormonal component? Also since ergotamine is a vasoconstrictor drug, is there a risk that it will make permanent damage from cerebral ischaemia more likely?

Focal neurological events should always be taken seriously and demand a full assessment, not just hollow reassurance.

As always, the history is of great discriminating value. Cerebral vascular disease is often a multifactorial problem and one can relax to some extent if the patient has no other adverse risk factors whatever. However, there would be concern if the patient were hypertensive, a smoker, already with a history of vascular disease, for example myocardial infarction or intermittent claudication, and there would also be concern about a bad family history of vascular disease whether it was from hypertension, diabetes or hyperlipidaemia. It would be reassuring if the patient had had focal neurological symptoms since early adult life with no residua.

Focal attacks which occur only on one side and have never ever occurred on the other may be due to a structural lesion such as an angioma, but if the episodes have clearly occurred on either side, then the cause of an important underlying structural disease is less likely. Sometimes sensory symptoms are only one-sided, but the visual accompaniment may clearly involve the visual fields from both cerebral hemispheres. The presence of headache is unusual for a thrombotic cerebrovascular event, but can occur. In focal epilepsy, there is often a march of the sensory symptoms and the other accompaniments of migraine are usually absent.

Many things are wrongly attributed to the menopause, but there is no doubt that some women have severe exacerbations of their migraine at this time. After the menopause, many women have far less trouble with migraine than during their reproductive years. However, those that are put on to oestrogen replacement therapy may have troublesome migraine as a result.

How you advise the patient would depend to some extent on the findings on examination. If the patient was in atrial fibrillation or had hypertension or a cardiac or carotid bruit, one would be suspicious that there was more to this than just a migraine attack. Furthermore, migraine victims are unfortunately not immune from tumours and they might have persisting neurological signs, including subtle changes in higher cortical function or even papilloedema.

Probably some basic investigations are indicated in all cases including urine and blood sugars, full blood count, including platelet count and sedimentation rate, and ECG and chest X-ray. If focal epilepsy is even a remote possibility, then an EEG should be performed. In some cases, it is reassuring not only to you, but to the patient, to have a normal CT scan. More rarely, it would be necessary to perform digital subtraction angiography.

Although ergotamine is a vasoconstrictor drug, there is no convincing evidence that giving it causes an exacerbation of cerebral ischaemia. Indeed there are good reasons to support its use, first for symptomatic relief and secondly because, in cerebral ischaemia, the use of a vasoconstricting drug is more likely to be effective on the normal intracranial blood vessels rather than those in the affected area. The former will therefore constrict with a tendency to divert blood to the area of most need.

The menopausal woman with migraine is often a most difficult management problem. It may be necessary to assess the whole lifestyle. All women should be advised to avoid excesses of physical and mental fatigue, they should eat regularly, but avoid those foods and drinks which are likely to aggravate their migraine. They should ensure adequate sleep. Some women will have to come off hormone replacement therapy.

For the treatment of the acute attack, since this patient likes ergotamine, I would continue using it. However she might gain benefit from changing its form of presentation. Some achieve considerable relief using an ergotamine inhaler. Others prefer it by rectal suppository or sublingually. An antiemetic such as metoclopramide or prochlorperazine can be very helpful in the acute attack.

If she has not yet used sumatriptan by mouth, I would advise trying it. She might find that, for her, it is the one antimigraine agent that is more effective than ergotamine. Sumatriptan and ergotamine should not be used in the same attack. Sumatriptan injection is licensed in migraine both with and without aura. The recommendation is not to give actually during aura as it will not prevent the oncoming headache.

For prophylaxis, it is worth trying aspirin if it is tolerated. It has the advantage of some antiplatelet activity which would have the effect of preventing hemiplegic migraine becoming complicated (i.e. the migraine attack leaving permanent signs). The usual prophylactic agents can be tried such as clonidine, pizotifen, β-blockers, calcium antagonists (although the author has rarely found these very useful in migraine) and, in this particular age group, antidepressants might be tried with good effect.

It is always worth keeping such patients under review and stressing that they should notify you if any change should occur in the nature of their neurological symptoms.

Sometimes, patients taking ergotamine are hardly ever free of headache but once they stop taking the drug the headache can get even worse ('rebound headache'), thus encouraging them to take even more of the same. These patients often need hospital admission where they can be transferred to a migraine prophylactic and sumatriptan.

Question 28.   Arteritis – don't be fooled by the ESR

A 65-year-old man complains of a right-sided headache of recent onset; on examination you find some scalp tenderness. His ESR comes back at 20. What do you advise?

This man may have cranial arteritis. Don't be put off by the normal ESR! He may need high dose steroid treatment to prevent sudden blindness.

If you have any doubt, therefore, refer to an appropriate clinic. A temporal artery biopsy might be required to confirm the diagnosis. Approximately 20% of patients with a cranial arteritis have an ESR within the normal range! Apart from the local arterial tenderness look out for jaw claudication – a pain which develops in the side of the face on chewing, particularly meat.

If you are happy about the diagnosis, high dose steroid therapy (i.e. 60 mg enteric-coated prednisolone daily) plus ranitidine should be started as soon as possible. If the patient fails to have relief of the head pain within 24 hours, then the diagnosis of cranial arteritis is unlikely to be correct and the steroid treatment can thereafter be withdrawn. Unfortunately, a number of conditions other than cranial arteritis respond to steroid therapy, for example migraine and cerebral and cranial metastases and therefore accurate diagnosis is necessary.

Once the patient has been well established on steroids, i.e. after 4 or 5 days, there is unlikely to be sudden irreversible visual loss. The dose of prednisolone can be reduced gradually over the first 2 weeks down to 40 mg a day and then reduced further over the following months. It is much more satisfactory to use the patient's symptoms as a guide to further reduction in steroid therapy rather than changes in the ESR. The recurrence of head pain and scalp tenderness would necessitate restoring the previously effective dose and then waiting for another month or two before attempting further reduction.

The arteritis tends to burn itself out more quickly in some patients than in others. It may be necessary to maintain a dose of 10 mg/day for up to 6 months and then to attempt reducing at say 1 mg/month.

Head injury

Question 29.   All through the night – observing head injury

A boy of 6 is playing on a climbing frame; he falls, bangs his head and is unconscious for a few seconds. He then cries and seems to make a complete recovery. What action should be taken? Are there any circumstances in which you would advise the parents to wake the child at intervals at night to make sure that he was only in normal sleep?

- The child should be admitted to hospital for observation.
- If this is not possible, unless the injury was very early in the day, the child should be woken at hourly intervals during the following night and the parents acquainted with the early signs of neurological deterioration.

The concern here is that the child is going to go on to develop a damaging or even fatal intracranial haematoma. Climbing frames are often 'strategically' placed over a concrete base and if the child doesn't hit his head on one of the horizontal bars as he falls, he does so on the concrete. Loss of consciousness, even if temporary, indicates a significant head injury. If consciousness is recovered quickly, it means that the brain stem injury was slight but, at the moment of impact, an intracranial vessel may have been damaged which may continue to bleed slowly over the next few hours. Temporal injuries by injuring the middle meningeal artery are particularly liable to do this and produce an expanding extradural haematoma. Facial and occipital blows are much less likely to produce the complication.

The physical features of an extradural collection are very minimal initially. Once they develop, the neurological decline accelerates and there may be very sudden deterioration with sudden intracranial pressure shifts. After the lucid interval, the child may start to complain of headache, anorexia, nausea and may vomit. He may become irritable, lethargic and then drowsy. Urgent expert assessment with CT scanning is indicated. A normal skull X-ray is of no reassurance. The onset of diplopia, unilateral pupillary dilation and hemisensory or motor features are ominous signs and a tentorial pressure cone is then imminent and, if the child is not in a neurosurgical unit by this stage, the outcome is poor. Obviously a susceptible child can suffer a focal migraine after injury giving all the above features (including a dilated pupil) but one must never accept this diagnosis without full assessment.

You will be well advised to refer any child who has been knocked unconscious to hospital for observation. If you do decide to keep the child at home and something goes wrong, you would be in an indefensible position legally. If the child is going to be managed at home, either because of parental insistence or because the hospital refused admission, then it is appropriate for the parents to get up every hour during the night to ensure that the boy is sleeping normally, rather than unconscious. This obviously requires waking the boy up to ensure that there is an appropriate response. This is particularly necessary if the injury occurred in the late afternoon or evening. If the injury was early in the day and the child was perfectly normal at bedtime, then there is relatively little danger.

The parents should be warned to let you know immediately if, after a lucid interval, there is any neurological deterioration (headache, vomiting, lethargy, diplopia or drowsiness). At this stage, prompt referral to the nearest neurosurgical centre (without the potentially dangerous detour to the local casualty department) is what I would do for my own child.

Unfortunately, many parts of the country have no readily accessible neurosurgical departments. Under these circumstances, refer promptly to one of your local accident surgeons with neurosurgical experience (you should know who has). You could give 4 mg dexamethasone intravenously or intramuscularly to the child before sending him in. There is NO time for delay once the child is 'going off'.

Question 30.   Minor event, major outcome

It is said that it is rare for there to be an important intracerebral complication from a head injury unless the patient has been knocked out. Is this true?

NO. The loss of consciousness at the time of a head injury implies that the brain stem reticular activating system has been temporarily damaged. It is possible to have cerebral hemisphere damage, damage to cerebral blood vessels or veins in the subdural space or one of the extradural arteries without sufficient disruption of brain stem function to produce unconsciousness.

Question 31.   Post-traumatic syndrome – fact or fable?

A man aged 40 years sustains a fairly minor head injury. For a considerable time afterwards he complains of dizzy spells, loss of concentration and irritability. A diagnosis of 'post-traumatic syndrome' is made. His doctor suspects that either the man is making much of it for purposes of compensation or else he is not made of 'the right stuff'. Might this be an unfair assessment? Is there a sound structural basis for the continuing symptoms?

- The post-traumatic syndrome does exist.
- Sometimes it can occur after fairly minor head injuries.
- It has a physical basis.
- It may occur in genuine, normally robust individuals who are highly motivated to return to work or play for whom the symptoms are a major inconvenience and where there are no thoughts of compensation.
- Clearly the symptoms might have more impact on those with a suspect pre-morbid personality, particularly when the injury occurred through no fault of their own and there are thoughts of compensation.

The main clinical features of the post-traumatic syndrome are:

- Headache: this is fairly typical of muscular-contraction headache, tends to get worse towards the late morning or afternoon and is made worse by noise. Particularly irritating, it seems, are other people's radios or televisions and small children playing.
- Mood changes, especially irritability and depression.
- Difficulty with concentration, particularly when there is any noise. The patient often says he cannot concentrate on more than one thing at a time and then only for short intervals.
- Poor memory: in patients with relatively trivial head injury, poor memory is usually a result of poor concentration.
- Vertigo: there is often a momentary feeling of dysequilibrium, sometimes with a rotary component, that comes on with sudden change of position. Not infrequently, it occurs on lying down or turning over on one side or trying to get up from bed. The lesion causing the feelings of dysequilibrium is thought to be a peripheral one in the inner ear rather than one in the brain stem. Usually it clears up within a month or two but in a few cases is more persistent.

If there is a background of headaches prior to the accident, then it is more likely that the headaches following the accident will be more severe, more frequent and persist for longer. If there is a history of depression or lack of drive, these features may be particularly troublesome. Similarly a person subject to vertigo may have the symptoms disproportionately worsened.

In the medicolegal area, however, this state of affairs could provide a field day for the lazy and greedy who will, of course, be attracted by thoughts of compensation. There is no doubt that, even in the most genuine cases, the protracted legal proceedings that often follow road or traffic accidents make a major contribution to the severity and duration of symptoms. Some patients must be regarded with suspicion. But even in those without any thoughts of compensation, symptoms may persist for up to 2 years. What is the physical basis for this condition?

The CT brain scan in such cases is normal. The changes in the brain are thought to be at a microscopic level. There are billions of tiny connections between the neurones in addition to the large main-line axons. The shearing stress produced by certain head injuries is thought to sever many of these tiny connections. For this reason, it may take many months, if not years, for the individual to feel his brain is working normally again.

Genuine patients may be helped by an explanation of what has gone wrong and reassurance that spontaneous recovery WILL occur. A combination of an antidepressant with fairly regular analgesia will make the patient feel better and more comfortable. If dizziness is a particular problem, cinnarizine is helpful, but if it continues to be a persistent feature, some re-evaluation of the case might be necessary to exclude previously undiagnosed brain stem involvement.

The patient should be protected from undue stress and strain until natural recovery has occurred. Although a period off work is often advisable, the previously disabled patient will often make a sudden and dramatic recovery for no discernible reason and ask to go back to his job.

If legal action is to be taken, the doctor should encourage the legal profession to arrange compensation as soon as possible.

Vertigo

Question 32. Dizziness gone; nystagmus remains

An otherwise healthy man aged 35 years has an episode of unexplained vertigo lasting nearly 3 weeks. He eventually appears to make a complete recovery. On examination, however, he still has nystagmus. What is the likely significance? How would you assess and manage the patient?

- In the absence of other neurological signs, it is likely that the patient has had some viral involvement of the inner ear.
- The persistence of nystagmus implies that the lesion has not fully resolved.
- It is necessary to attempt to exclude other causes.

Few symptoms cause more distress than vertigo. Patients feel wretched, nauseated and often vomit. Yet vertigo is only rarely due to anything sinister. It may prove difficult to convince the sufferer that such dramatic symptoms may be due to small lesions of little pathological significance because he felt that he was dying. The patient usually expects the doctor to be most interested and sympathetic, perhaps to do a lot of investigations and then to treat the condition satisfactorily. He is likely to be disappointed and need fairly subtle handling.

Vertigo may be produced by a lesion situated anywhere along either the right or left vestibular pathway starting from the inner ear (labyrinthitis) to the eighth nerve (vestibular neuronitis) to the cerebellopontine angle, the brain stem and then up to the temporal lobe. In an attempt to localize the site of a patient's problem, it is usually necessary to seek other features, because often the description of dizziness doesn't help. Diplopia and facial numbness would imply that the lesion was in the brain stem. Deafness and tinnitus would be in favour of a peripheral lesion involving the inner ear. If the patient loses consciousness or has disturbed consciousness during the attacks of vertigo, then a temporal lobe lesion is likely.

The causes of vestibular pathway damage are varied. An over-simplification is that in the young, it is viral and, in the old, it is vascular. Both bacterial and viral infections of the middle and inner ear may be implicated. Many cases are post-traumatic. The patient might be in an early stage of Menière's disease. To make this diagnosis, it is usually necessary to follow the patient over an interval to document recurrent episodes and accompanying features of tinnitus and progressive deafness. A plaque of demyelination due to multiple sclerosis in the brain stem is not an uncommon cause of vertigo in young and middle-aged individuals. Very rarely neoplasms may present in this way. It is exceptional for tumours to do so without there being any other physical manifestation.

Clearly one needs to determine whether there is: any deafness or tinnitus; a past history of middle ear disease; any recent trauma or infection particularly diarrhoea. The enteroviruses are frequently responsible. A past history of neurological disease should be tactfully sought including retrobulbar neuritis and attacks of sensory disturbance. A history of migraine, as in this case, and travel sickness indicate that the patient will be far less tolerant of feelings of vertigo than other individuals.

On examining the patient, the presence of nystagmus after the symptoms of vertigo have resolved would imply that there is persisting vestibular pathway damage for which the patient has now compensated. It doesn't help distinguish which type of lesion has been responsible for the vertigo unless the nystagmus is of a particular variety. Vertical and rotatory nystagmus occur with central lesions. Ataxic nystagmus is almost invariably due to an intrinsic lesion in the brain stem. In this condition on looking to the right, for example, the left eye fails to adduct normally, the right eye can abduct but, in abduction, demonstrates florid nystagmus.

If a patient continues to demonstrate an ataxia without continuing to feel vertigo, then the lesion was probably central rather than peripheral. The ears should be examined and in addition the facial and corneal sensation tested. In the elderly, a blood pressure difference between the two arms and a subclavian or vertebral artery bruit should be sought.

Investigations of the patient with vertigo are usually not required unless there are clear pointers from the assessment. Looking for viral antibodies is usually a waste of time in this context. If there is any suspicion that the patient might have multiple sclerosis, then it would be reasonable to arrange an MRI brain scan and possibly a CSF examination.

In managing such a patient, it is usually wise to warn that it is possible that there might be a minor relapse some weeks hence and the Driving Licence Authority will require the patient to be off driving for at least 6 weeks free from paroxyms of vertigo. Once the patient is asymptomatic, treatment with drugs is usually not indicated, but patients are often reassured if they are given a small supply of 25 mg prochlorperazine suppositories to keep by them to take at the very first sign of any further trouble.

Patients with a past history of travel sickness or migraine very often tolerate vertigo extremely poorly and make up a substantial portion of the patients who keep returning to the surgery complaining bitterly about their symptoms of dysequilibrium. These patients may respond more satisfactorily to a drug used in migraine prophylaxis such as propranolol or pizotifen than the more conventional antivertiginous agents such as cinnarizine or prochlorperazine.

If there are no more signs of neurological disturbance in the patient mentioned, the most likely diagnosis is a viral involvement of the inner ear. In patients over 60 years, although viral vestibular damage is still a common cause, the possibility that symptoms are due to vertebrobasilar ischaemia needs to be considered.

Question 33.   Giddiness in the elderly

An elderly man gets giddy when he turns his head suddenly. Is the cause more likely to be labyrinthine or vertebrobasilar in origin? How would you treat labyrinthine symptoms in such a patient?

Despite popular belief, if an elderly patient experiences sudden feelings of rotatory vertigo, coming on immediately on movement of the neck, it is most likely to be labyrinthine in origin and is not likely to imply recurrent vertebrobasilar ischaemic attacks. (For further information see Question 71.)

Probably the best medication for elderly patients with labyrinthine problems is cinnarizine. The advised adult dose is 2×15 mg tablets three times a day. This can make many people sleepy and often one or even half a tablet, two or three times a day, will suffice.

An MRI brain scan is very sensitive to the presence of ischaemic lesions and posterior fossa tumours. With the reassurance of a normal scan many patients, and their relatives, are easier to manage.

Multiple sclerosis

Question 34.   Retrobulbar neuritis

A female secretary aged 20 years has an attack of retrobulbar neuritis. How likely is this to have been caused by multiple sclerosis? How would you manage such a case?

- Multiple sclerosis is the most likely cause of retrobulbar neuritis in a woman of 20 but by no means the only one.
- I would avoid the approach of an ophthalmic registrar who said to a patient 'I would like you to go along to a neurologist to see if this is the first sign of multiple sclerosis'. Such a referral makes management a little difficult!

The causes of retrobulbar neuritis are:

- Multiple sclerosis.
- Herpes zoster.
- AIDS.
- Syphilis.
- Sinusitis.
- In children following mumps, measles, chickenpox or infectious mononucleosis.

However, most cases of retrobulbar neuritis in adults are caused by multiple sclerosis. The figures given for the chance of an individual with retrobulbar neuritis going on to develop multiple sclerosis (MS) vary considerably between series from 30% to 75%. It is the presenting symptom in approximately 15–20% of patients with MS and most patients with MS (80–90%) will show some evidence of an attack of optic neuritis at some stage. The chance of progression is influenced by age, male sex, the presence of HLA DR2, winter onset, any sign of relapse, or the CSF showing an oligoclonal pattern on electrophoresis and multiple lesions on magnetic resonance imaging.

When faced with a patient who has virtually gone blind in one eye and who has severe pain on eye movement, it is not fair to burden them with the worry that this may be the first sign of a feared disease. They have enough concern about the sudden deterioration in the vision and the fear that they might go blind permanently. They need reassurance that there will almost certainly be a reasonable recovery of vision on that side. Over 90% of individuals improve to 6/12 vision, i.e. that required by Licensing Authorities for driving a car.

It is exceptional for retrobulbar neuritis to occur simultaneously on the two sides. When it does so, the prognosis is clearly not so good and those with late-onset retrobulbar neuritis bilaterally have poor prognosis for vision. However, the vast majority of patients can be strongly reassured that they are not going to go blind.

Since retrobulbar neuritis is the presenting feature in only 15–20% of MS patients, a large number of patients will already have had neurological symptoms although they might not have been so noteworthy as a painful sudden loss of vision. When taking details of the past medical history, one can tactfully ask about previous neurological symptoms like diplopia, vertigo, balancing or sensory difficulties and, on examination, there may be hints of disordered eye movements, some problem with vision on the other side and abnormal coordination or abnormal reflexes and disturbed sensation. If other neurological features are discovered, then the chance of a patient with retrobulbar neuritis having multiple sclerosis is very high.

In the past it has been my practice to do very little in the way of investigation in the type of case described above unless, or until, another attack develops (see Question 36). It now appears, however, that 70% of retrobulbar neuritis patients show MRI evidence of demyelination and with the development of beta-interferon (see Question 37) the advantage of early diagnosis of MS may lead to all patients with retrobulbar neuritis having an MRI scan as a routine.

Question 35. Prognostic pointers in multiple sclerosis

A diagnosis of multiple sclerosis has been made in a young man. He comes to the surgery in a state of high agitation because of the delay in confirming the diagnosis. He wants to know the prognosis in as far as it can be given. What are the features of his disease that might give you cause for optimism or pessimism?

The prognosis in multiple sclerosis is extremely variable.

It depends to some extent on the immune status of the individual but luck also plays a very major part. For example a plaque in the white matter of the frontal lobe may produce no obvious neurological difficulty, whereas a plaque of similar size in the cervical spinal cord would have a devastating effect on mobility and sensation.

The most reliable prognosis in MS can be given only after about 5 years from the first symptom. The relapse rate tends to be highest in the first few years. Patients do better if there are long intervals between attacks (relapsing remitting MS), if they make good recovery after every relapse and if they have predominantly sensory symptoms. One can be optimistic at 5 years if a patient has little significant handicap. It should be emphasized to newly diagnosed patients that at least 85% of patients with multiple sclerosis are able to lead reasonably independent lives and it is only the unlucky minority, who become severely handicapped, that give the disease a bad name.

Men who present with a motor onset in middle life tend to do badly. They often show a chronic progressive variety of the disease right from the start (primary progressive MS). There are some patients who start off with a relapsing remitting disease, but convert to a chronic progressive variety (secondary progressive MS).

There is much variation. I have seen individuals who have had little trouble for 20 years and then within 6 months are in a wheelchair and others who have several relapses in quick succession shortly after presentation and then no further trouble for many years. The 'lesion load' on MRI scanning is of some value in predicting prognosis but it still pays to be as optimistic as possible with every patient, particularly as beta-interferon becomes available (see Question 37).

Question 36. Demyelination confirmed

A 28-year-old woman whose mother has MS has developed numbness in a leg. This is how her mother's problem started! How should she be managed? How reliable are brain scanning, CSF examination and various electrical tests at excluding the possibility of multiple sclerosis?

First, evidence is now available indicating that there are genetic influences on MS development. Without MS in the family the chance of developing it is 1:800. If one first degree relative has the condition the risk rises up to 5%. If both parents are affected the risk to the children is 7%. She may be worried not only about herself, but about the possibility of her own children going on to develop the disease.

A careful history and clinical examination may give the answer. The cause of her sensory disturbance may well be a peripheral problem in the leg, such as a lateral popliteal lesion or more commonly an L5 or S1 dermatome sensory disturbance. If the ankle jerk is absent, the patient can be told emphatically that this does not occur in multiple sclerosis which is a central nervous system disease.

You will usually find that the patient will want to be examined not only by yourself, but by a 'specialist'. Even if nothing is found on examination, the patient should perhaps be offered investigation. Many will decline with the reassurance of a normal examination, but others with temperaments preferring to know rather than not know, will want to have investigations.

Unfortunately, conventional X-ray CT scanning is of little reassurance. Many MS patients will have perfectly normal CT scans. Magnetic resonance imaging (MRI scanning) is very much more powerful. It is extremely sensitive at picking up plaques of demyelination. Over 95% of patients with MS will have areas of abnormal signal detectable in the brain or spinal cord. This is the best single test for multiple sclerosis and, fortunately, becoming more readily available. The MRI scan has to be taken in context, because multiple vascular lesions can have similar appearances, but clearly at the age of 28, multiple sclerosis is very much more likely as a cause for scattered areas of abnormal signal.

Cerebrospinal fluid examination may be abnormal in over 85% of patients with clinically definite multiple sclerosis. It is necessary to perform electrophoresis of the CSF proteins. The typical finding is an elevated IgG_4 and IgG_5 – an oligoclonal pattern. If this is present with no similar abnormal bands in the serum, then it can be taken that the immunoglobulins are being generated in the CNS and again, in context, multiple sclerosis may be the reason for the abnormality.

The three electrical tests are visual evoked potentials (VEPs), auditory evoked potentials and somatosensory evoked potentials. The principles are the same. The patient has a stimulus and the conduction time is measured. In VEPs, for example, the time taken for a visual stimulus to reach the occipital visual cortex is measured. VEPs are the single most useful electrical test. They are positive in over 80% of patients with clinically definite multiple sclerosis. There doesn't have to be a past history of retrobulbar neuritis. In fact, the test is more useful when it is positive without a past history. An abnormal VEP will then highlight an unexpected second lesion in the visual system which may be well away from the site of immediate clinical interest indicating that the neurological problem is multifocal.

Auditory evoked potentials are slightly less powerful. Possibly around 60–70% may be positive in confirmed cases and somatosensory evoked potentials have similar pick-up rates.

A combination of all three evoked potential studies being negative and a normal CSF would be very reassuring that the patient did not have multiple sclerosis.

Question 37. New hope in MS?

Two patients come into a GP's surgery. The first is a 23-year-old girl with a recent attack of optic neuritis (resolving) and a vague history of a few previous sensory disturbances. A report from the neurologist says that her MRI scan shows several small white matter lesions. The second is a 50-year-old man with progressive MS who is now virtually confined to a wheelchair but able to continue working as a lawyer. Is either likely to benefit from beta-interferon?

Beta-interferon is the first form of treatment in MS which has been shown to slow down the rate of progression of the disease. Understandably this 'breakthrough' has been over-reported and expectations may be inappropriate and too high.

As yet, no results are available from the ongoing trials in chronic progressive MS. In summary, the following has been shown in relapsing remitting MS:

- Beta-interferon reduces the number of relapses during follow-up by about 30% compared to placebo.
- Beta-interferon similarly reduces the number of new lesions developing on MRI during follow-up.
- More recent results are encouraging re the development of further disability during follow-up.

However, beta-interferon does not improve disability caused by previous attacks.

So on present evidence the young woman should be considered for beta-interferon treatment although she might feel that the inconveniences caused, so far, hardly justify frequent, regular injections. The lawyer, on the other hand, will have to be encouraged to be patient pending the results of the on-going trials of his type of MS – something he may be reluctant to accept.

Question 38. Treating with steroids

A man of 25 has short episodes related to his multiple sclerosis every 6 months or so. These attacks resolve quickly on ACTH. Is this common and should ACTH be used in all such circumstances?

No! The majority of patients appear to have some beneficial response to steroids in their first few attacks only. Later they are not so sure and it is just a minority of patients who continue to derive consistent benefit from subsequent courses of steroids. It is only in these patients where it is reasonable to continue to give steroids. Even then, they should be confined to short courses started promptly at the first sign of a relapse.

There is no satisfactory evidence that ACTH is any better than oral steroid therapy. Injections, of course, have a much stronger placebo effect than tablets and every doctor can provide an anecdote of a patient who responds better to injections of ACTH than to oral prednisolone.

There is reasonable evidence now that in a severe relapse it is worth trying a course of high dosage methylprednisolone intravenously daily for 5 days. This seems to be effective at improving the rate of recovery in some cases. It certainly should not be used for mild relapses but where patients have suddenly become severely affected, it should be tried. Whether the promising results from the pilot studies will be confirmed by larger clinical trials remains to be seen.

In patients with MS, steroids probably reduce the time to recovery from a relapse, but they do not affect the extent of recovery. Indeed if the patient turns out to be extremely steroid responsive, then the diagnosis of MS should be questioned. He may turn out to have another condition such as a connective tissue disorder which is masquerading as multiple sclerosis.

Certainly the doctor should not push on prescribing steroids when there is no evidence that they are producing any physical benefit, except a psychological one. Patients with MS are more vulnerable to steroid complications and less dangerous 'placebos' are available, e.g. vitamin B_{12}.

Question 39. Motherhood and MS – recipe for disaster?

Does pregnancy tend to make multiple sclerosis worse, better or have no effect? When a young MS victim asks if she should become pregnant, what do you advise? 'Is MS hereditary?' she asks. How do you reply?

- Although many women with MS sail through pregnancy without any problem, others may suffer a severe relapse either during pregnancy or during the puerperium.
- Pregnancy should only be advised if a woman is really desperate for a child and has a realistic chance of being able to look after it.
- There is a slightly increased risk that one of the children may have the condition.

There are considerable changes in a mother's immunological system during pregnancy. These may influence the body's immune defences against multiple sclerosis and a relapse may occur either in pregnancy or shortly afterwards. There is no reliable way to predict what will happen.

A relatively mild case with little disability may have quite a severe relapse and thereafter be disabled. The mother may then blame the child for rendering her paraplegic and incontinent.

Conversely, more severe cases may go through pregnancy with no problems whatever. In the case of handicapped women, it is important to discuss with them their ability to look after a young child. The wife's assessment may be quite different from that of the husband and the rest of the family.

There is no specific contraindication to the woman having an epidural anaesthetic to help delivery. Caesarean section, like all other operations, should be avoided if possible to reduce the chances of a relapse resulting from it.

An invariable question is whether multiple sclerosis is inherited. Unfortunately there does seem to be a genetic component. Her children will each have up to a 5% chance of developing MS.

Question 40.   MS and the Pill

A young woman aged 24 years with multiple sclerosis asks whether it is safe for her to go on oral contraceptives. How should she be advised?

There is no contraindication to the oral contraceptive pill up to the age of 35, but after that, other forms of avoiding pregnancy may need to be discussed. Many women sensibly choose sterilization.

It is probably unwise for the doctor to suggest the possibility of the husband having a vasectomy. At some stage, the husband may wish to remarry, either because his wife is dead, or because he has been unable to cope any longer with having a disabled wife.

There is no convincing contraindication to older women with MS taking hormone replacement therapy.

Question 41.   Surgery best avoided

A woman of 35 with multiple sclerosis who walks with the aid of a stick has troublesome varicose veins. How should she be advised with regard to surgery?

Some patients with MS seem to have a relapse of their condition after surgery. This occurs more often than can be attributed to the play of chance alone; probably the surgical trauma acts as an immunological trigger and relapse may be generated. It is not possible to predict which patient will have trouble postoperatively; patients who have previously relapsed in these circumstances should be treated very cautiously.

All surgery in patients with multiple sclerosis should be questioned. Only really important operations should be performed. Cosmetic operations should be avoided. The patient might be asked how he or she would feel if the operation caused a relapse. Often the answer clarifies the course of action. Surgical colleagues very often are not aware that a relapse occurs because it may do so after the patient has been discharged from hospital and after the first outpatient review appointment.

Tremor and parkinsonism

Question 42.   The shaking hands – benign familial tremor

A woman of 40 is embarrassed by her tremor. She has been told that it is benign familial tremor. Can anything be done about this? Is there any association with Parkinson's disease? Is it an indicator of poor general health?

- Social tricks can be employed to help in this embarrassing but harmless condition. Drugs, such as propranolol, might also be of some use.
- There is no association between familial tremor and Parkinson's disease.
- It is not an indicator of poor health. On the contrary!

Although the GP can exclude other pathological conditions such as hyperthyroidism, it is usually worth referring such patients to a neurologist for confirmation of the diagnosis (Table 3).

Patients can be advised to use tricks such as resting the hand on the furniture. Alcohol often relieves the tremor but can lead to dependence. Propranolol from 10 mg to 40 mg up to four times a day can be useful. Occasionally small doses of primidone or diazepam may help. Patients should be warned to avoid cigarettes and coffee. Bronchodilators can make the condition worse as can heavy work, vibrating machinery and anxiety.

In many cases, all that is required is reassurance. It should be emphasized that they are not going to become handicapped. After having gone through the various drugs available, some patients accept that as long as it is nothing serious, they can put up with it. They are cheered by the thought that benign essential tremor is one of the few conditions that may be associated with a longer than normal life expectancy!

Table 3

Tremor	Parkinson's disease	Familial tremor	Cerebellar syndromes
At rest	+++	0	0
Maintaining a posture	++	+++	+
With intention	+	+	+++

Question 43.   Parkinson protocol
Is there a conventional protocol for treating the average case of Parkinson's disease?

No. First, ask whether the patient needs any therapy at all. Many patients with mild parkinsonism, particularly the elderly, do not need any drug therapy, and just need to be kept under observation with therapy introduced at a later stage if necessary.

It is important to resist the temptation to treat the patient, particularly the elderly patient, too vigorously. One should emphasize that drugs are used to help control symptoms so that they can just cope with day-to-day existence. The drugs are not used in an attempt to make the patient perfectly normal again. If one attempts to abolish the symptoms completely, the chance of side effects is increased very substantially.

For some people, treatment should begin with a small dose of levodopa (50 mg) combined with either carbidopa 12.5 mg or benserazide 12.5 mg. This should be taken after food initially to avoid nausea. Later on when the patient is used to the drug, extra doses can be introduced between meals without nausea in most people. The plan should be to give small doses regularly. As time goes by, it may be necessary to reduce the interval between doses to just 2-hourly. The new controlled-release preparations of levodopa may be helpful in smoothing out the therapeutic effect and many neurologists now advise using C/R therapy at the outset. Effort should be made to try to avoid using a high dose three times a day; this is very likely to give a kick to begin with which the patient might appreciate, but eventually he will run into trouble with peak dose dyskinesias and troublesome on/off effect. Some advanced patients, however, choose to return to three big doses per day so that, at least, they can get something done for a short while.

Small doses of bromocriptine, or another direct dopamine agonist, spread throughout the day, may help to limit the marked fluctuations in levodopa therapy. Another way of smoothing out the levodopa effect during the day is to use the monoamine oxidase B inhibitor – selegiline 5 mg a day. Sometimes selegiline can have a mildly antidepressant effect. There is now concern about an apparent, unexplained, increase of mortality on the combination of selegiline and levodopa and some patients choose to omit selegiline.

Question 44.   Anticholinergics and bromocriptine
Under what circumstances in the treatment of Parkinson's disease would you use an anticholinergic or bromocriptine?

Anticholinergic
The anticholinergic drugs can be useful in treating parkinsonism, especially in controlling tremor and rigidity; they are also helpful in reducing

hypersalivation. The problem is their side effects. The tendencies to produce urinary retention in men with prostatism, to increase intraocular pressure in those prone to glaucoma and to produce drying of the mouth are well recognized. However, the main problem in using them is the confusion they can produce, particularly in the elderly. Some neurologists do not use them in elderly patients at all, others confine their use to patients who are under 75, others to under 65. Patients' responses are somewhat unpredictable. In a patient whose parkinsonism is badly controlled by other means, it is often worth trying a small dose of an anticholinergic and warning the relatives and the patient that they should be on the look-out for any tendency to get 'muddled'.

Bromocriptine
Bromocriptine is a direct dopamine agonist – others are pergolide and lysuride – and may be helpful in treating some patients with Parkinson's disease. Its main side effects are nausea and postural hypotension. At one stage, it was suggested as a possible monotherapy for parkinsonism, starting off with a low dose and it was suggested that there might have been delayed beneficial effect after, say, 3 months on low dose therapy. However, it is now rarely used on its own, but in combination with levodopa treatment. It helps to smooth out the effect of therapy so that there is less of an on/off experience, it also permits a lower dose of levodopa to be used and hence the patient may be spared some of the troublesome side effects.

Note: Bromocriptine's other main indication in neurology is in the treatment of prolactinomas. In the female it inhibits galactorrhoea and restores menstruation and, in the male, corrects impotence. It is so efficient in the inhibition of these tumours that often surgery is avoided even when the lesion has expanded beyond the pituitary fossa.

Question 45.   Confused by drugs?
A man of 69 on antiparkinsonian drugs suddenly becomes confused. Is it more likely that the drugs are responsible for this confusion rather than some other factors?

- One of the drugs that he is taking is a likely cause. The anticholinergics are particularly prone to produce confusion.
- Other causes of toxic confusion state should be considered.

Parkinson's disease is unfortunately one of the causes of dementia. Although some patients may retain normal intellect many years after developing the disease, the addition of an anticholinergic drug may push someone with subclinical dementia into being severely disorientated and confused. Otherwise normal healthy elderly people may develop a toxic confusional state if given an anticholinergic drug (see Question 44).

Amantadine is well known to produce quite florid and sometimes unpleasant nightmares and should be stopped in susceptible patients. Levodopa itself can also cause confusion and the dose may have to be reduced in some patients and in others it may even have to be stopped. A wife often finds it easier to cope with a sensible but immobile husband than with one who is hypomanic and mobile.

Such an episode of confusion should be the right moment for reconsidering the patient's therapy. Pruning any unnecessary drugs and maintaining just a very small dose of a levodopa preparation may be optimal. Parkinsonian patients are particularly prone to polypharmacy.

The possibility of an intercurrent infection should be considered, usually of the urine, sometimes of the chest. One should ask about the possibility of a head injury, sustained in one of the inevitable falls. Also chronic painful conditions, either physical or emotional, may lead to such a state.

Question 46.   Octogenarian Don Juan

An elderly gentleman of 80 takes a levodopa product for his parkinsonism; no other treatment controls his symptoms satisfactorily. The management at the local day centre he attends complains because the man has started to embarrass the old ladies he encounters by asking sexual favours and making provocative gestures. How does one proceed?

Try cyproterone acetate.

When levodopa therapy was first used, the story spread quickly that old men in geriatric institutions were suddenly rediscovering their libido and chasing the nurses. Levodopa was tipped as an aphrodisiac. Sadly this is not the response when the drug is used in normal individuals!

In patients with Parkinson's disease who are imprisoned and frustrated by the rigidity and bradykinesia, the improved mobility produced by using the drug allowed them to do what they had been longing to do for ages. This is what seems to have been the case in most individuals. However, in a minority, there is little doubt that libido is significantly increased and most neurologists have come across wives who have refused to allow their husband to have the drug for these sexual reasons. Others of course are delighted!

First, one should ask whether an anti-parkinsonian drug is needed at all and, in mild cases, the levodopa can be removed without any significant reduction in his mobility. Amantadine or possibly an anticholinergic drug could be tried, watching for side effects of confusion and hallucinations. However, if levodopa is the only agent that produces a satisfactory response as in this case, then it is cruel not to treat his parkinsonism. The increased libido that results from the drug can be blocked by giving cyproterone acetate.

Question 47. Parkinson pills and dyspeptic distress

A woman of 65 with relatively severe Parkinson's disease has a long history of hiatus hernia and duodenal ulceration; she feels that most drugs upset her. What do you advise?

- Check that she is not taking metoclopramide for her hiatus hernia as it could make the Parkinson's disease worse.
- Tell her to take her medication in smaller doses spread through the day.

Patients with severe Parkinson's disease will normally accept side effects for symptomatic relief of their extrapyramidal problems. At her age, and with her sensitivities, it is probably not worth trying an anticholinergic, certainly not as a first-line drug. One would do better to concentrate on a levodopa preparation and one can reassure the patient that if there is a side effect it is likely to be nausea, and by introducing it at low dosage in combination with an extracerebral decarboxylase inhibitor (e.g. levodopa with either benserazide or carbidopa) patients can tolerate it quite well. It is only a very small proportion of patients who cannot take levodopa when introduced to it correctly.

Nausea can be limited by taking the drug after food; this doesn't mean a full three course meal, but in most cases a cup of tea, a biscuit or a slice of toast will suffice. In very sensitive patients, nausea can be controlled further by taking 10 mg domperidone half an hour before the levodopa preparation.

Adequate blockage of the extracerebral decarboxylase requires 75 mg of carbidopa or benserazide in most patients. This means giving combined pills, containing levodopa 50 mg, up to 6 times a day (breakfast, coffee, lunch, tea, supper, late night drink) or, if appropriate, two such pills three times a day.

If the patient cannot tolerate levodopa, then she might achieve relief from amantadine hydrochloride taken as 100 mg twice daily. The therapeutic effect of amantadine in parkinsonism is unfortunately temporary in the majority of patients, lasting no more than a few months, but in others the therapeutic effect seems to be present for some years.

Question 48.   The shaking limb – levodopa overdose

A wife of a patient with parkinsonism who is on levodopa therapy contacts you to say that her husband has developed uncontrollable involuntary movements of one limb. Is this the result of the disease, or the treatment? What should be done?

- These involuntary movements are almost certainly due to the levodopa therapy. They imply that too much of the drug is available at certain times of the day.
- The dose needs to be reduced and redistributed throughout the day.

Involuntary movements, often writhing in nature, are a common side effect of levodopa therapy. The face, mouth and tongue may be involved or any of the four limbs in combination. Many patients on levodopa are susceptible to peaks and troughs of the drug at various times during the day. The involuntary movements often come on within an hour or so of taking a dose of levodopa.

Levodopa therapy nowadays is often started in general practice and unfortunately it is not uncommon for patients to be given the larger tablet or capsule size at the outset. Patients should never start with a dose as high as 100 or 250 mg. Side effects can often be reduced or avoided by the very gradual introduction of levodopa therapy beginning with tablets containing 50 mg of levodopa once a day with food to avoid nausea. The frequency is then gradually increased so that the patient has a tablet with breakfast, coffee, lunch, tea, supper and at bed time. This ensures a more uniform level of the drug throughout the day. This can be improved further by the addition of the monoamine oxidase B inhibitor, selegiline, but there are safety concerns now about this combination (see Question 43).

Some patients with these writhing dystonic movements resulting from an excess of levodopa therapy may resent the reduction in the dosage because they miss the 'lift' of the surge in levodopa levels after, for example, a large 250 mg dose. Patients often tolerate the most extreme involuntary movements, which may produce bruising, and say they are quite happy to put up with such disturbances if it permits them to be released for at least a time from the imprisonment of their rigidity.

Much misery is caused by unrealistic expectations of both the family and the patient with parkinsonism. One should emphasize early in the disease that the aim is to attempt to control symptoms. We are not attempting to eradicate them altogether. If the latter is attempted, then side effects are inevitable sooner rather than later. There is often some resentment on the patient's part and it sometimes helps to be open with them and to say things like: 'You don't come into my surgery blaming me for not curing your baldness and grey hair, so why blame me for not curing your parkinsonism'. This may seem harsh, but when put across in the right tone, the air is cleared and the patient may be happier and easier to manage in the long run.

Question 49.   Phenothiazines or parkinsonism?

A woman of 50 years with a history of endogenous depression has done well on a tricyclic/phenothiazine combination tablet which she has taken for several years. Unfortunately, she doesn't respond as favourably to tricyclics alone and when she ceases her medication, she becomes unacceptably depressed. She begins to develop a coarse parkinsonian tremor. Should she continue her present medication and be given something such as benzhexol in addition? Would continuing the treatment cause permanent damage to the basal ganglia?

The patient probably has Parkinson's disease and not just a phenothiazine reaction, because if the patient has marked tremor, it is extremely unlikely to be just due to the phenothiazine. On these drugs, it is rigidity and bradykinesia that are predominant and not tremor. What you are probably seeing is a patient with idiopathic parkinsonism who is having her symptoms aggravated by the drugs.

There is some evidence that prolonged phenothiazine drugs may lead to permanent basal ganglia damage. Even when the drugs have been stopped, some of the extrapyramidal symptoms may persist, although they are usually less marked than when the patient is taking the drug. You should therefore consult a psychiatrist and ask him/her if there is any other antidepressant, for example a tetracyclic or even a monoamine oxidase inhibitor which the patient may try, because clearly it is preferable to avoid the phenothiazine if at all possible.

Usually an anticholinergic is an acceptable way of countering the extrapyramidal side effects when phenothiazine treatment is essential. If no other antidepressant is acceptable in this patient, then an anticholinergic might be tried and hopefully it will not lead to confusion of hallucinations. Unfortunately, levodopa therapy tends to be disastrous when used in patients who need phenothiazines for psychiatric reasons. It makes any tendency to psychosis much worse.

Note: Levodopa should not be prescribed with a monoamine oxidase A inhibitor.

Question 50.   The damsel's distressing dystonia

A girl of 17 has postoperative vomiting following a minor operation. She is given a phenothiazine and develops a dystonic crisis. You advise her not to take any more phenothiazines for the time being. How long do you advise this restriction to continue?

She is very unlikely to get another attack, in similar circumstances, after the age of 20.

Some sort of dystonic reaction may be observed in up to 5% of patients on a phenothiazine. Often it occurs after the first dose. In my experience, the most commonly implicated drug is metoclopramide. Fortunately, severe reactions are rare. When they do occur, they are very frightening, particularly when in a child who cannot explain what is going on. Children are perhaps vulnerable because the dose of phenothiazine used is not quite appropriate for their sensitive and responsive basal ganglia. They often demonstrate marked opisthotonos and may have an oculogyric crisis. Onlookers may think the child is having a fit or has developed meningitis with marked neck retraction.

It is somethat unusual for a girl as old as 17 to have a dystonic reaction but of course not impossible. The author has never seen a severe case in someone over the age of 20 as a result of a single perioperative dose of an antiemetic phenothiazine.

Phenothiazines block dopamine in the basal ganglia; there is a balance between this compound and acetylcholine. The blockage of dopamine results in a relative excess of acetylcholine. The attacks normally respond very satisfactorily to an anticholinergic drug. For a severe reaction, the drug should be given parenterally and two forms are available, either procyclidine or benztropine.

The patient should be reassured that if a phenothiazine is necessary in future for vomiting, a dystonic reaction is much less likely to occur, especially once the patient has reached the age of 20. For further reassurance, the patient might be offered the choice of having some prophylactic procyclidine or benztropine for further elective procedures.

Cerebrovascular problems

Question 51.   Fit and healthy with a carotid bruit

An apparently fit and healthy man aged 58 has been for an expensive medical check-up. You are notified that he has a bruit over the left carotid artery. What action should you take?

- Carotid bruits are a common incidental finding. The more you look, the more you will observe.
- The patient should not be frightened to death with talk of 'blocked artery to the brain and the need for urgent investigation'. A large percentage come to no harm.
- Unless there were other circulatory risk factors (see below) I would not worry him with it, suggest no further investigation and advise him to take an enteric-coated aspirin three times a week.

The chances are that the bruit is due to a stenosis at the carotid bifurcation, but there are other possibilities. The carotid may be kinked. It may be due to high flow because the patient is nervous. Anaemia or thyrotoxicosis may be responsible.

In a patient who has had no cerebral symptoms and continues to have none, the risk of cerebrovascular problems is quite small provided the patient has no other important risk factors for vascular disease, i.e. hypertension, smoking, hyperlipidaemia, diabetes, polycythaemia.

So, without worrying the patient, it is important to determine whether any of these important circulatory risk factors exist. He should be asked about symptoms of angina, peripheral vascular disease and transient retinal or cerebral ischaemia. An ECG, full blood count, blood sugar and blood cholesterol will already have been done at the recent medical. If all the above are reassuring, then it could be safely assumed that he was in a low-risk group and I would be tempted not to worry him with the thought that he had a threatening carotid stenosis. I would just advise him to take one enteric-coated aspirin on alternate days as a good preventative measure for men over 50 years.

If he is in a high-risk group, i.e. with more than one vascular risk factor, then he should be investigated further. It is just as important to look at the heart as it is to look at the head because carotid stenosis may represent a more generalized vascular problem. He might need both a neurological and cardiological opinion. The investigations might include Doppler assessment of the carotid arteries, MRI scan and MRI angiogram. Also relevant may be stress test, echocardiography and coronary angiography.

In symptomatic patients with over 70% stenosis, carotid endarterectomy reduces the risk of stroke by approximately 50%. Asymptomatic people with tight stenoses are also at risk from stroke, particularly if there are other risk factors. However, final results of endarterectomy trials in the asymptomatics are still awaited.

If a patient is found to have triple vessel coronary disease, or left main stem disease, then he may also need to have a coronary artery bypass graft. If not, the treatment should aim to improve risk factors by optimal control of blood pressure and blood sugar and to control the blood fats.

If the patient realizes that he has got a high cholesterol, he will want to try and do something about it even if at present there is no really convincing evidence that doing so necessarily improves the prognosis. Most patients should go on to aspirin if they can tolerate it. If not, then it can be suggested that they try using one of the fish oils, for example halibut liver oil. For the moment, I am unhappy about prescribing other antiplatelet agents like ticlopidine or dipyridamole as a preventative measure in asymptomatic patients.

Question 52.   Takes aspirin but still has transient ischaemic attacks

A man aged 65 who had two transient ischaemic attacks 6 months ago was started on aspirin. He presents with a further attack despite taking aspirin conscientiously. What action would you take?

The action to take in this particular case is:

● Urgent referral for further investigation.

A transient ischaemic attack (TIA) is a major pointer to impending cardiovascular problems. Within 2 years of having presented with a TIA, 14 out of 100 patients will have had a cerebrovascular accident, a myocardial infarct or be dead. In spite of this, it has been estimated that 19 out of 20 patients with transient ischaemic episodes do not get appropriate referral in the UK.

Unfortunately, many patients are either just cheerfully reassured that 'it was only a spasm' or are put on aspirin without any further investigation, although aspirin prevents only 3 of the 14 end-points mentioned above. This is an unacceptable state of affairs. All such patients should be properly assessed to see if anything else can be done.

The history is of major importance. If the attacks occur with sudden changes of position, for example on standing or turning, or when a patient remains standing after exercise, the cause might be haemodynamic rather than thromboembolic. Particularly vulnerable to this kind of attack are those receiving hypotensive or antianginal therapy. Transient monocular blindness on the same side as the involved hemisphere, however, suggests that the TIA is caused by emboli from the ipsilateral carotid artery.

Patients should be thoroughly examined for other evidence of vascular disease including hypertension, diabetes mellitus, myocardial ischaemia and peripheral vascular disease. Elevated blood pressure is a frequent accompaniment of a TIA. Many patients have cardiac arrhythmias, particularly atrial fibrillation. The presence of carotid or cardiac bruits will immediately focus attention on one of these sites.

Screening tests should include blood count to exclude polycythaemia and thrombocytosis, ESR to exclude an arteritis, blood sugar and lipids, a serobiological test for syphilis, urea and electrolytes, midstream specimen of urine, chest X-ray and ECG.

The heart should be examined in every case. If there is any cardiac bruit, atrial fibrillation or the patient is having bilateral episodes without evidence of carotid disease, echocardiography is indicated.

In most cases, the carotid arteries need to be investigated. Nowadays this can be done atraumatically using Doppler and MRI angiography. If there is any doubt digital subtraction angiography (DSA) may be necessary.

Although hypertension is the most important risk factor in people presenting with TIA, it should be handled with care and blood pressure reduced cautiously. Smoking and excessive alcohol intake should be discouraged. Diabetes should be optimally controlled as should gross hyperlipidaemia and obesity.

Of the clotting factors, fibrinogen is of particular interest nowadays. Fibrinogen level is raised by smoking, by infection or the presence of vascular disease. It is probably also raised by stress. There is some evidence that it can be lowered by the lipid-reducing agents, clofibrate and bezafibrate.

If aspirin has failed to prevent attacks and if there is a significant carotid stenosis, endarterectomy should be advised. If no surgically amenable leison has been found, then it is reasonable to use warfarin. Personal experience dictates that this generally underused drug can be very efficient in suppressing transient ischaemic attacks resistant to antiplatelet therapy. Perhaps at some time in the future, clinical trials will show that much smaller doses of warfarin than those generally used might have a most beneficial and safe action in the prevention of transient ischaemic attacks. Ticlopidine, an anti-platelet agent available on a named patient basis in the UK, may be tried if other measures fail.

Question 53.   Anticoagulants at 80?

A retired hospital matron aged 80, sharp in both mind and body, has two transient ischaemic attacks in one week. How would you proceed with investigation and treatment? Would you consider giving anticoagulants to a patient of this age?

This woman has a lot to lose. Don't be therapeutically nihilistic. Investigate as in Question 52. Remember, particularly, to check for arrhythmia, cranial arteritis, diabetes and hypertension. Treat the blood pressure if it is above 180 systolic but do not bring it down below 140 systolic.

Enteric-coated aspirin 300 mg on alternate day dosage and fish oil capsules, 4–6 a day, might be adequate but if anticoagulants are indicated because there is, for example, fibrillation or an embolic focus, warfarin should not be withheld. Ranitidine can be prescribed to protect the gastric lining; hypertension must be brought under control before the anticoagulant is started. Aim for a prothrombin ratio of 1.5–2 (not 2.5–3.5 as you would in a younger patient).

If medical treatment fails to prevent further transient ischaemic attacks and if there is a carotid bruit, then carotid surgery may be considered because the risks are justified. The patient should be referred for investigation; this should be non-invasive in the form of Doppler studies, MRA and intravenous DSA. If there is an amenable lesion and no evidence of impending myocardial infarction, then carotid endarterectomy may be recommended. It is not a major insult to the system if all goes well. The perioperative risk of stroke is somewhere in the region of 3–5%. Many old people sail through the operation and are discharged from the hospital 4–5 days afterwards. They should be maintained on the antiplatelet therapy postoperatively – a common omission.

Question 54. Bell's palsy or stroke?

A man of 73 who has had two small cerebrovascular accidents in the past appears to have developed a Bell's palsy. He does however seem to have some sensory changes on the side of the face. How could one distinguish Bell's palsy from a small CVA? Does it matter anyway?

Bell's palsy tends to be overdiagnosed. In the young, it is not uncommon for patients with multiple sclerosis to remember a bout of unilateral facial weakness. It was probably a small plaque of brain stem demyelination and not a Bell's palsy. In the elderly, the diagnosis is usually a cerebrovascular accident. In this patient, his age, his past vascular history and the presence of a sensory disturbance on one side of the face imply a vascular cause and it is not a Bell's palsy. Less commonly, facial weakness may result from a Ramsay Hunt syndrome with Herpes zoster involving the geniculate ganglion.

Bell's palsy is often preceded by a day or two of pain in the mastoid region (Table 4). Involvement of the forehead and eye closure are much more profound in a Bell's palsy than in upper motor neurone lesions.

Table 4

	Bell's	CVA
Preceding pain	+/–	–
Involvement of forehead	+++	+
Eye closure	Incomplete	Usually complete
Taste involved	+	–
Hyperacusis	+	–
Dysarthria	+	+
Sensory disturbance	–	+/–

Also in a Bell's palsy, taste and hyperacusis may be involved implying a peripheral cause for the trouble. You do not get these two findings in a patient with a central lesion, though both conditions will produce a dysarthria because of poor facial movement on the affected side. Sensory signs tend to be absent in Bell's palsy and tend to be present in most patients with a vascular event. The site of the cerebrovascular lesion is often the cerebral cortex; sometimes it is the brain stem. When it is the latter, there may be some diplopia as well as minor facial sensory change.

It IS important to get the diagnosis right. If it is a painful Bell's palsy, impressive symptomatic pain relief may follow oral steroid therapy. If it is a further small vascular event, then it becomes essential to reassess medication in order to try to prevent further such attacks. If one just ignores a series of minor cerebral events, patients will sooner or later develop a multi-infarct dementia or a major stroke. An MRI scan, therefore, is indicated to confirm or exclude brain stem lesions and others in clinically 'more silent' areas.

Question 55. Hypotensives after a cerebrovascular accident?

A man aged 71 years has quite a severe stroke leaving a speech difficulty and a right-sided hemiplegia; after 2 weeks he starts to make a gradual recovery. Prior to the stroke, he had taken β-blockers for his hypertension, but is now on no such medication. The GP records his blood pressure at 200/105. Should he restart treatment?

Yes, there is good evidence that treating blood pressure after stroke reduces the chance of recurrence and clearly the last thing this man wants is a further cerebral event to impede his recovery or to add to his handicap. The blood pressure should be treated cautiously introducing one agent at a low dose initially and the programme should be to attempt to reduce the pressure to the region of 160 mmHg systolic.

Where patients have carotid or vertebral artery stenosis, a slightly higher blood pressure than normal may be required in order to maintain cerebral blood flow in the face of arterial narrowing. One should watch carefully for symptoms of dizziness and faintness. These are likely to occur before symptoms of focal cerebral ischaemia as blood pressure falls. A higher systolic pressure, say in the region of 180 mmHg, may have to be accepted in such patients.

As a general policy, one does not treat raised blood pressure in the first 2 weeks after a stroke; this is because, in many cases, it is a compensatory response attempting to improve cerebral blood flow to deprived areas. One certainly would wish to treat those who have very severe sustained hypertension, say with a systolic pressure of over 220 mmHg, because, if left unmodified, this will lead to an increase in cerebral oedema within the first 10 days. Otherwise, the doctor leaves the blood pressure alone and only considers treating those patients who are still significantly hypertensive after 2 weeks.

Question 56.   Only a little unwell with a subarachnoid!

During the period of one month, a GP sees two cases of subarachnoid bleed, not as collapsed patients at home, but as mobile patients in the surgery. Is this uncommon? Apart from the obvious, classic case, what should you do if you suspect the possibility of a subarachnoid leak? Is it always easy to differentiate a subarachnoid from a migraine? Are the new, less invasive, angiographic methods revealing any more aneurysms?

- Sometimes symptoms from a subarachnoid leak are not particularly severe.
- If the possibility of a subarachnoid crosses your mind send the patient in for a lumbar puncture.
- There are similarities and differences between a subarachnoid and a migraine.
- The new intravenous angiographic methods may not reveal important small aneurysms.

The cardinal feature of a subarachnoid is that the headache comes on very suddenly and is usually severe. Usually! But is anything in medicine that simple? The first bleed need not be as severe as you would imagine.

In migraine, the headache tends to build up over a period of a few minutes and is nearly always better within 24 hours. After a subarachnoid the patient is often groggy for several days. It is very common to have a small 'herald' bleed a week or two before the catastrophic bleed. Try to refer patients then before it is too late.

Before a subarachnoid haemorrhage, some patients can remember a trickling sensation on one side of the head. Although photophobia and vomiting can be present in migraine, always look for a stiff neck and perform a Kernig's test in a patient with headache. In only rare cases is some stiffness of the neck absent in a subarachnoid. A third nerve palsy shows that the subarachnoid is very likely to have come from a berry aneurysm involving a posterior communicating artery.

Any patient with a sudden severe headache should be referred promptly. No one of any quality should mind seeing a patient immediately when the suggested diagnosis is a subarachnoid haemorrhage or meningitis. Unfortunately, the patient who might have had a 'herald' bleed often turns up at the outpatients more than 2 weeks after the episode. Lumbar puncture and scan will not then be able to rule out a haemorrhage and intra-arterial angiography will be necessary. Unfortunately, intravenous digital subtraction angiography, though adequate to show up carotid or vertebral artery blockage, is inadequate to exclude small or even medium size berry aneurysms.

Somewhat surprisingly, after a large subarachnoid leak, patients are not only at risk from further haemorrhage but also from damaging cerebral infarction. The latter is due to arterial 'spasm' in response to blood breakdown products in the subarachnoid space. This spasm may be relieved and infarct size reduced by using nimodipine, a calcium antagonist.

Dementia

Question 57. Huntington's disease – the dreaded legacy

A girl of 18 whose mother has Huntington's disease consults you on the likelihood of developing the disease herself. How accurate would the forecast from genetic counselling be? Should she be advised to be sterilized?

- An extremely accurate test is now available.
- The girl should be counselled before she has the test regarding all aspects of the future, including sterilization.

Huntington's disease is an autosomal dominant condition. For years it has been possible to tell a girl like this that she has a 1 in 2 chance of having the condition. It was a matter of waiting for a long time in the hope that signs would not develop. Now a genetic test is available which predicts, with over 95% accuracy, whether, or not, a person is going to develop the disease. The girl should be referred to a department of clinical genetics. Blood samples from other family members are no longer required. The genetic test can also be used to exclude Huntington's disease in some demented patients with involuntary movements.

Telling young people that they almost definitely have an awful, currently untreatable, progressive neurological disease has its serious repercussions. The girl should be counselled before she has the tests performed.

Perhaps you should not be telling her to be sterilized; this should be her decision when she is in full possession of the facts. If she is going to develop the disease, then sterilization would be quite reasonable, although she might prefer to await intrauterine diagnosis (and then the opportunity to abort any affected foetus).

Far more of a problem than the girl is the male who possibly has the disease. In the very early stages of its development, he may be disinhibited and more promiscuous than normal and there is evidence that such males produce more off-spring than average!

The impact of genetic counselling on the prevalence of Huntington's disease has been disappointing. An unacceptably large number of children are born to individuals at risk of developing the disease. GPs, neurologists, psychiatrists and geneticists need to do better and, hopefully, the accurate genetic test now available will have a dramatic effect.

Question 58. 'Am I losing my mind?'

A woman aged 56 comes to her doctor and says that she is afraid that she is developing pre-senile dementia. Her mother had it and was hospitalized permanently from the age of 55. Could she be right or would insight go before symptoms become apparent?

- Most pathological conditions producing dementia, including most cases of Alzheimer's disease, are not, on present evidence, usually inherited.
- Although it is possible for people to have insight into what seems like a decrease in mental ability, anxiety or depression rather than dementia might well be the cause.
- Assessment and reassessment at intervals should be carried out to see if there is actual loss of cerebral function.

It is often said that most dementing patients are brought to the attention of the doctor by their family. The patients tend to cover up their deficiencies and those who present themselves are, in most instances, suffering from anxiety state which produces poor concentration and, as a result, poor memory. Like all generalizations, this is of limited value and it is not always the case.

Reassurance without assessment, therefore, is of little value and if there is a possibility of dementia the patient should be referred to a neurologist. Intelligent patients, in particular, can be aware that something is happening and should be taken seriously. It is not uncommon for patients with a family history of Huntington's disease to commit suicide when they notice signs of the disease developing in themselves.

Question 59. Reversible dementia

What proportion of patients with apparent dementia have a reversible cause?

The proportion of patients with a reversible cause will depend to a large extent on the pattern of referral of the demented population studied.

- Of those referred to a neurological unit, which would tend to exclude the patients who are very elderly, about 15% were found to have a remedial cause. This is an extremely good yield for what is otherwise a serious and progressive condition.
- One would expect only a small proportion of those referred to a geriatrician to have a treatable cause.

Brain failure nearly always merits expert assessment. It is important to get as accurate a diagnosis as possible in order to predict prognosis and to guide management. It may turn out that the patient is not demented at all, but has psuedo-dementia from depression.

Some patients turn out to have a toxic confusional state, where sudden disorientation occurs in the context of an infection or severe pain, medication or injury. There is a need to be guarded about the prognosis in these patients because very often the patient does, in fact, have early mild dementia and temporarily decompensates as a result of infection, for example. False assurance might be given: 'just toxic confusion'. Some spontaneous recovery can also occur in patients with multi-infarct dementia.

Otherwise dementia tends to be steadily progressive and it is very difficult to keep the patient's relatives on the doctor's side if an accurate diagnosis has not been attempted in the face of relentless deterioration.

Question 60.   Alzheimer's or a vascular dementia, or both?

Is there a significant difference between the clinical features and prognosis of Alzheimer-type dementia and a vascular dementia? How do the treatments differ?

- There are significant differences between the onset and prognosis of Alzheimer's disease and multi-infarct dementia, a common form of vascular dementia.
- There is no treatment presently available for Alzheimer's disease.
- The treatment of vascular dementia will depend upon the cause as revealed by investigation and may be rewarding.

Approximately 85% of dementias, whether senile or pre-senile, are either Alzheimer's disease, multi-infarct dementia or a mixture of the two. Alzheimer's disease is four times as common as multi-infarct dementia, about 20% of cases being of mixed aetiology. In the older Alzheimer patients, about 40% will show cerebrovascular changes. The rarer forms of vascular dementias need not be discussed here.

It is possible to be reasonably sure about which dementia a patient has from the use of a simple 'ischaemia score' (Table 5). A score of 6 or more implies vascular dementia. A score of 4 or less implies a primary degenerative dementia (like Alzheimer's disease). Patients with mixed dementia (a combination of Alzheimer's disease and multi-infarct dementia) may be misclassified initially. MRI scanning is extremely valuable in diagnosis.

The onset of multi-infarct dementia is usually sudden – in contrast to the gradual development of cortical failure in patients with Alzheimer's disease. However, patients with Alzheimer's disease may appear to

Table 5 Ischaemic score

Feature	Score
Abrupt onset	2
Stepwise deterioration	1
Fluctuating course	2
Nocturnal confusion	1
Relative preservation of personality	1
Depression	1
Somatic complaints	1
Emotional incontinence	1
History of hypertension	1
History of strokes	2
Evidence of associated atherosclerosis	1
Focal neurological symptoms	2
Focal neurological signs	2

Total 6 or more: probably vascular dementia
Total 4 or less: probably Alzheimer's
Some cases are mixed!

present suddenly. There may, for example, be a very sudden deterioration as a result of an intercurrent infection. Alternatively, their dementia may be rapidly revealed by the illness or demise of a spouse who has been protecting and supporting the patient for months or years.

Focal signs are much more likely to be found in patients with vascular or mixed dementia. In the early stages of the disease, the finding of dysphasia, visual disturbance or focal motor or sensory signs would be strong pointers to vascular dementia.

The prognosis in the two conditions is considerably different. In Alzheimer's disease, there tends to be a steadily progressive deterioration, whereas in multi-infarct dementia, there is often a stepwise deterioration with a reduction in abilities occurring at the time of an infarct, with some recovery taking place before another infarct causes further deterioration and so on.

It is clearly very important to attempt to analyse the problem in a patient with multi-infarct dementia as soon as possible to prevent further damage occurring. One may find that the patient has a cardiac source for emboli. Observation that the patient is in atrial fibrillation, even intermittent atrial fibrillation, is extremely important, because anticoagulants may produce very substantial improvement. This depends, of course, on there being no medical contraindications and the presence of a carer who can administer the drug reliably. Some patients may be found to have severe carotid stenosis in which case surgery may prevent further emboli.

Hypertensive and diabetic problems should be detected and treated appropriately, occasionally with considerable benefit.

On the assumption that many infarcts are thromboembolic in origin, patients are often put on antiplatelet therapy. There is no definite evidence that this is of value in preventing decline in multi-infarct dementia, but the first author's opinion is that it should be tried until further evidence is available.

There is no satisfactory drug treatment as yet for preventing deterioration in Alzheimer's disease. The memory problems of Alzheimer's may be linked with problems of neurochemical synthesis in the cholinergic system. Anticholinergic drugs are known to make confusion very much worse and research is afoot for suitable, palatable and effective cholinergic medication.

The prime carer should be considered and sometimes it is necessary to give the patient night sedatives in order to allow the carer to get some sleep. In the later stages of the disease, psychotropic drugs may be required temporarily to control disinhibited and unacceptable behaviour.

The long-term prognosis in dementia is clearly poor. Some cases can be kept at home by caring families for several years, but eventually institutional care in a psychiatric or psychogeriatric ward is required. The prognosis for survival from the time of onset is clearly much shorter in the elderly but, with an ageing population, the implications, as far as the number of psychogeriatric beds are concerned, have not been faced realistically.

Question 61.   'It's not worth investigating at his age!'

A usually fit and agile old gentleman aged 84 has, in the opinion of his family, become 'very odd' over the past few weeks. 'His mind has gone, doctor' they say with resignation. At what age would you NOT consider investigating dementia?

- I would thoroughly investigate patients below the age of 75 who develop dementia.
- After the patient has passed 75, the investigations I would carry out would depend more on the general physical condition than the date of birth.
- I would not investigate an extremely old patient, of poor general condition, with a long history of gradual deterioration.

Whatever the age of the patient, I would think it worth looking at the full blood count, urea and electrolytes, the liver function tests, the serum vitamin B_{12}, the thyroid function and the syphilis serology. I would make sure that a toxic confusional state due to drugs or infection is excluded. Any history of headache or head injury associated with the dementia would warrant a CT scan to exclude a subdural haematoma.

Acute onset dementia has a better prognosis than one of chronic onset and enough cases turn out to be reversible to make investigation worthwhile.

Question 62.   Do cerebrovasodilators have a place?

Is it worthwhile giving patients with dementia some kind of vasodilator in the hope that it might improve the cerebral blood flow?

There is no convincing evidence that vasodilators work. Nevertheless, there is occasional anecdotal material suggesting that improvement can take place and as the products are relatively harmless they could be tried, especially if the family expect a therapeutic gesture.

Try to determine the cause of the dementia and manage accordingly. A better option, in a non-specific case, would be to use an antiplatelet such as aspirin (in an effort to prevent cerebral microinfarction). Sometimes antidepressants can be surprisingly effective when depression is compounding the cognitive efficiency.

Depression, which might be producing a pseudo-dementia, can lift really quite quickly and spontaneously even without any antidepressant treatment. The mother of a close friend, for example, had been depressed and retarded for months. She then fell and fractured her hip and had an immediate recovery from her depression – the medical equivalent of 'kicking the television'.

Question 63.   Benign dysmnesic something-or-other

A rather worried man phones up the surgery to say that a doctor something-or-other at the hospital told him that he had benign dysmnesic syndrome. He wants to know what it is. Explanation please.

Everyone knows, or thinks he knows, what amnesia is: dysmnesia means a partial disturbance of memory rather than a complete loss (compare the subtle English distinction between dysphasia and aphasia which is not recognized by our American cousins!). Dysmnesia is a helpful word that is not used enough.

Some deterioration in memory affects most people over the age of 18. It becomes particularly marked once over the age of 70, but difficulty remembering people's names is quite common in otherwise normal people in middle age and is not necessarily a sign of impending dementia. However, the concern a doctor should have when presented with a patient who is complaining of deteriorating memory is that there is a distinct possibility that the patient is in the early stages of dementia and I would have the greatest misgivings about reassuring such a case without more information, particularly reassessment following a period of observation.

Only a neurologist or psychiatrist would label a patient as suffering from a benign dysmnesic syndrome. Presumably the diagnosis has been made on the grounds that the memory defect is still mild, despite several years having lapsed since the first sign of a memory disturbance was noted.

Alternatively, a patient may have a moderate memory problem, but no other evidence of any intellectual decline on careful psychometric testing.

Reassurance after a single superficial assessment without detailed psychometry is of no value. Remember that one of the most common causes of poor memory is anxiety sometimes mixed with depression, where a patient does not concentrate and, without adequate concentration, memory is inefficient.

Most patients in their 50s and 60s who have minor memory problems, essentially centred about forgetting names, have this benign dysmnesic syndrome – of reassurance to most of us!

Weakness, fatigue and narcolepsy

Question 64.   Motor neurone disease – any grounds for optimism?

A man aged 60 is told that he has motor neurone disease. 'Oh dear!' he says in horror, 'that's what David Niven died of, wasn't it doctor?' Is there any variation of development of the disease that might allow for some small amount of optimism?

There are no grounds for optimism. The main hope would be that the diagnosis was incorrect. Every patient with suspected motor neurone disease (MND) deserves an expert neurological opinion.

Occasionally a patient with a spinal muscular atrophy is misdiagnosed as having motor neurone disease. This condition tends to have a much more benign prognosis, especially if it is focal, for example with the weakness and wasting affecting essentially one limb or side and no accompanying upper motor neurone signs.

As an approximate guide, patients with only lower motor neurone signs, i.e wasting, fasciculation and weakness, may survive for up to 10 years from the onset of symptoms.

Once upper motor neurone features develop with brisker reflexes and extensor plantar responses, the prognosis is less than 5 years. Once bulbar symptoms develop, death is usually within 18 months.

The patient can, usually, be reassured if all that is found is a few fasciculations in muscles that are normally strong. All that is advised in this situation is to keep the patient under observation and, if any weakness or other features develop, to refer to a neurologist subsequently.

Two new forms of treatment, insulin growth factor and riluzole, may improve survival but have little demonstrated benefit on disability.

Question 65.   Fasciculation – when not to worry

Fasciculations are a common finding in a GP surgery in apparently fit individuals. Under what circumstances should it be taken seriously as a probable indication of motor neurone disease?

I see about one medical student a month with fasciculations who thinks that he has motor neurone disease but he invariably has 'benign fasciculations'. Fasciculations in the calf are extremely common and are usually of no concern. This is probably because L5/S1 discs with S1 nerve root irritation are very common, particularly in sportsmen; usually there is no need for any action. Little twitching movements of the eyelids (benign myokymia) also deserve reassurance. It is also frequent for patients to complain of little twitches in one of the small muscles of the hands, for example, the thenar eminence and the thumb may actually move as a result, usually when the patient is at rest. Again these are usually benign. Fasciculations are also common in other muscles when resting after exercise. This may be particularly so in the convalescence phase of some viral infection.

An ominous combination is when you find fasciculation in the limbs when there is wasting and weakness and where the reflexes are abnormally brisk. This usually means a combination of an upper and lower motor neurone problem and motor neurone disease is then a distinct possibility. The youngest patient I have seen with it was 18!

Question 66.   ME or not ME? – that is the question

A 35-year-old psychiatric nurse with a good previous work record is trying to run a home and still work full-time. She presents complaining of exhaustion and being tired all the time. She thinks that she has myalgic encephalomyelitis (the ME syndrome), having read about it in the paper. How should she be advised?

- She should be investigated for other causes of fatigue.
- She should be given time off work until recovery occurs.

Some of my neurological and psychiatric colleagues dispute the existence of the ME syndrome. I do not and believe that some highly motivated individuals are genuinely affected.

Myalgic encephalomyelitis (the ME syndrome) is a fashionable diagnosis. Perhaps a better term is the 'post-viral fatigue syndrome' – in the USA, it is known as the TATT syndrome (tired all the time!). Most patients are self-diagnosed. The ME Society has indulged in a lot of publicity recently. Many suggestible people, if they read about any condition, immediately think they have got it.

Fatigue is very common after viral infections, particularly those which produce some myalgia during the acute phase of the illness. The vast majority of patients recover spontaneously within just a few weeks. Why then, do some patients continue to have symptoms? It is now thought that, in a minority of these, there is virus infection persisting which their immune system is unable to eradicate normally.

Of those who continue to complain over a period of some months, some are undoubtedly neurasthenic individuals who cannot cope with the normal pace of life. Others are generally depressed. Some may have serious neurological disease such as multiple sclerosis where fatigue may be an irritating, persisting symptom after the more focal neurological symptoms have been forgotten. Other patients may have genuine muscle disease, like polymyositis.

What clinical features are helpful?

A good pre-morbid personality is very reassuring and some patients who were previously very energetic seem to be genuinely frustrated by not being able to get up and do the things they really want to do. The cardinal feature is that the patient's activities are limited by muscle pain and fatigue, even on relatively minimal exercise like walking a few yards. The sort of patient who can actually walk a couple of miles and then says he is exhausted afterwards has not got the ME syndrome. The patients are not actually weak when tested. If for some reason an ME patient has to push himself for an important commitment one day, then he usually is completely exhausted the next.

There is usually some interference with higher cortical function. The patients do not have the same mental stamina as previously, they often have difficulty concentrating and may have word-finding problems – minimal nominal dysphasia.

How should the patient be handled?

They should be told that there is no miracle drug treatment and that they shouldn't go in for crank diets or treatment such as anti-yeast therapy with nystatin. There is no evidence that this is helpful at all.

Amantadine seems to help improve energy in some sufferers, as do the more stimulating anti-depressants e.g. imipramine, but this tends to throw even more of a question mark over the aetiology of the condition.

They should be advised against exposure to other virus infections wherever possible and perhaps should avoid travel to areas where gut viruses are common and they should be careful to avoid the types of food where they are most likely to develop gastrointestinal upsets.

If they get another viral infection, they are likely to suffer a setback.

They should be encouraged to expect spontaneous recovery and, while waiting for it to occur, they should 'pace themselves'.

In this particular instance of somebody trying to run a home and a full-time job, the patient should just accept that all she should do for the moment is to manage as best she can with running the home and to give up the job. Usually, in genuine cases, this decision will have been made by the patient already and if the patient has been able to do both jobs, then one could be fairly sure that she has not got the ME syndrome.

Question 67.   The woman who couldn't get out of her chair

A woman aged 64, over a fairly short period, finds difficulty in getting out of her chair and walking upstairs. From what kind of condition is she most likely to be suffering? Should she be referred if she were 84?

- She is most probably suffering from a proximal muscle weakness.
- Yes, if she were 84, she should still be referred.

Difficulty getting up from a chair implies a weakness of the proximal muscles. The cause is usually a muscular disorder once the more obvious problems like severe arthritis and gross obesity, which should be clinically obvious, have been excluded. Neurologists are normally delighted to see patients with proximal weakness because they are an interesting group and often one can do much to help the acquired varieties.

At this age, with short history, a dystrophy (i.e. an inherited muscle disease) is unlikely. An inflammatory cause is quite likely. Has the patient any pain? If so, she might have polymyalgia rheumatica or polymyositis.

Metabolic causes are common, the most common being dysthyroid muscle disease, usually as a result of hyperthyroidism. Hypokalaemia and, very occasionally, hyperkalaemia may be responsible. Similarly, hypo- or hypercalcaemia may be responsible. Patients with Cushing's syndrome often have proximal muscle weakness.

Many drugs can produce muscle weakness, especially the corticosteroids, the diuretics (by producing hypokalaemia) and penicillamine, by producing a myasthenia gravis-like disease. The patient may have a serious underlying disease like a bronchogenic carcinoma.

A few patients may have a neuromuscular junction problem, either myasthenia gravis or the myasthenic syndrome (the Eaton–Lambert syndrome – usually from an underlying bronchial carcinoma or a connective tissue disorder).

Samson's weakness is now thought to have been the Eaton–Lambert syndrome associated with a connective tissue disorder – also causing alopecia. The only common neuropathy which presents with a predominantly proximal weakness is the Guillain–Barré syndrome and this will need to be considered.

Clearly, an accurate diagnosis is well worth making and generally the sooner the patient is seen the better. Many patients can be sorted out by a few simple blood tests, notably: thyroid function tests, electrolytes, calcium, creatine phosphokinase, ESR. A minority may need to go on to have electromyography and possibly a muscle biopsy under local anaesthetic.

Question 68.   Narcolepsy or tired out?

A housewife brings her 45-year-old husband to see a GP complaining that all he does when he gets home from work is to go to sleep. Is this one end of the normal spectrum or is there something wrong? Would any treatment help?

He might well have something wrong with him, for example narcolepsy, which should respond well to treatment.

First, the severity of the problem should be ascertained: is it that he just falls asleep after supper in front of the TV after an exhausting day at work, while she is still fresh from a less demanding day at home? Or does he feel sleepy at other times?

A narcoleptic will often have shown signs of needing more sleep than normal from his teens or early 20s. Sometimes there is a family history. The narcoleptic will often fall asleep during a meal.

He often goes straight into rapid eye movement sleep rather than slow wave sleep and he might fall face forward into food. It is not uncommon for him to fall asleep during conversations and on the telephone. It is frightening when sudden somnolence occurs at the wheel of a car and irritating for the passenger when it occurs on public transport, resulting in missing his stop. The patients nearly always sleep extremely well at night and when they wake from sleep, they are refreshed. There may be associated features, in particular a form of cataplexy where muscle tone suddenly drops as a result of sudden emotion or laughter. Patients may also have sleep paralysis where they wake and are quite unable to move until someone touches them. They also, associated with this phenomenon of going into rapid eye movement sleep, have hypnagogic hallucinations.

If you suspect narcolepsy refer to a neurologist as the patient should have an EEG and possibly a CT scan to exclude a hypothalamic lesion. Treatment with long-term dexamphetamine is usually required.

A patient has not got narcolepsy if he sleeps badly at night and then catches up during the day. Remember the possibility of the sleep apnoea syndrome in patients who are overweight with a short neck and who snore heavily.

Spinal problems

Question 69.   Don't manipulate the neck!

Many people with stiff neck have their necks manipulated by an osteopath or even a medical or orthopaedic practitioner. The technique, accompanied as it so often is by a series of popping and cracking noises from the spine, frequently produces sudden and considerable relief. Apart from those cases with real instability of the atlantoaxial joint as occurs in rheumatoid arthritis, or where there is bone pathology such as secondary deposits, is this procedure potentially dangerous?

Yes. Every neurologist will have seen somebody who has had damage to one of the vertebral arteries at the time of manipulation which has gone on to produce a vertebrobasilar territory ischaemic event. Much more frequent than this, however, is nerve root damage. It is only occasionally that the spinal cord is injured. The degenerative changes in the joints and soft tissues of the neck may be aggravated by manipulation, although temporarily the pain may be eased.

Osteopaths and other manipulators have an unrealistic idea of how frequently they run into trouble with cervical manipulation. The reason for this is that patients often feel a little guilty about having gone to them and, when something happens, they tend to take part of the blame themselves and they don't go back to complain to the osteopath.

In cervical manipulation, when popping and cracking noises occur, the manipulator is not putting 'discs back'; it is a trick analogous to finger cracking. However, there is no doubt that in selected cases it can be helpful in reducing the duration of periods of neck pain.

Pain in the neck, of almost any cause, will result in an increase in muscle tone which attempts to limit neck movement, thereby avoiding increasing the pain further. This increase in muscle tension is often on one side, an abnormal posture is assumed, usually a scoliosis and a loss of lordosis and, after muscle tension has been maintained for a while, the muscle begins to hurt.

After a few days, the protective effect of the muscle tension in reducing movement may no longer be necessary, but the bad habit has been learned and some local treatment at that stage may be most helpful in reducing the muscle spasm thereby reducing the secondary pain.

Violent wrenching of the spine is not indicated; usually local treatment with massage and gentle repositioning, sometimes with traction, are all that are required to accelerate spontaneous recovery. Some are helped by a temporary collar.

Patients who are particularly at risk from cervical spine manipulation, apart from those mentioned in the question, are those who have atheroma in the cervical and vertebral arteries. These individuals may suffer damage to the endothelium during manipulation and, on the area of damage, a thrombus may form and later occlude one of the vertebral arteries or break off and embolize into the vertebrobasilar tree.

Nerve root injuries are much more likely to occur when the patient already has nerve root symptoms in one of the arms in addition to the neck pain. You should warn these patients actively against manipulation. Well-trained osteopaths would not dream of advising manipulation under these circumstances, but the patient might be unfortunate and find his way to a less scrupulous practitioner.

Question 70.   Stiff neck, bad mornings

A man of 74 has had a headache for over 6 months, worse in the mornings. Apart from a stiff neck, there are no other abnormal findings on examination. An X-ray shows a moderately severe degree of cervical spondylosis. How likely is this to be the cause of his symptoms?

Cervical spondylosis is an extremely common cause for neck pain and restriction of movement. Sometimes it is the cause of a chronic headache, usually occipital, but it may be generalized. Frequently the pain is worse in the early morning. This is thought to be the result of less spontaneous movement of the head and neck at night. Sleeping in one awkward position for too long irritates the worn joints in the neck and generates secondary muscle spasm and pain.

The main causes for early morning headaches are:

- Hangover.
- Raised intracranial pressure from cerebral tumour or intracranial haemorrhage, or severe hypertension.
- Depression.
- Cervical spondylosis.
- Cranial arteritis.

The history and examination will help you decide which of these is the most likely explanation in this man. A 6-month history is against it being neoplastic, but remember that neck flexion may be restricted in patients with posterior fossa tumours where the cerebellar tonsils are pushed down through the foramen magnum – flexion of the neck produces irritation and is therefore resisted. Often in cervical spondylosis there is a restriction, not only of flexion of the neck, but also of lateral rotation and, to some extent, extension. Testing for scalp tenderness is not emphasized in some medical schools and many doctors examining patients for headache will not feel the scalp to find if there are any tender spots. One should never forget the possibility of a cranial arteritis in elderly people with headache and an ESR should be performed in every case. The patient's temperature should be checked. Headache is such a common longstanding symptom that one is at risk from delaying diagnosis of, for example, meningitis in a longstanding headache sufferer.

Management of neck pain
Often altering the pillows and arranging that the patient wears a soft collar at night, and if necessary a firm collar during the day, will produce considerable relief, both in the neck and head pains. Some patients also need the support of an anti-inflammatory analgesic, often best taken in the evening or at night. To reduce gastrointestinal upsets, the anti-inflammatory drug can be given by suppository, e.g. an indomethacin suppository.

Question 71.   Stiff neck, dizzy head

A man of 68, who has known cervical spondylosis, complains of bouts of vertigo. Are these most probably vertebrobasilar in origin? How likely is it that a patient with cervical spondylosis will have vertebrobasilar ischaemia?

- The vertigo is more likely to be vestibular.
- Cervical spondylosis and vertebrobasilar disease frequently coexist without being connected. Cervical spondylosis does not cause vertigo.

It is a very common misconception that, because a patient has cervical spondylosis and also neurological symptoms, the two are connected. Cervical spondylosis is common in middle and old age. Vertebrobasilar symptoms are very common over the age of 70, therefore it is not infrequent for the two problems to coexist in the same individual – but are they causally linked? Probably but not very often!

The suggestion that the patient has vertebrobasilar symptoms is usually made when he/she complains of sudden dizziness on change of position, usually involving some head and neck movement. The cause for this immediate feeling of dysequilibrium is usually a pre-existing vestibular system lesion on one side; it is often peripheral in origin in the labyrinth and nothing to do with the cervical spondylosis or vascular disease. It very rarely implies a vertebrobasilar ischaemic attack and statistically it would be very unusual for such a thing to occur every time a patient moved his neck in a certain position but not in others. For example the patient may be able to turn to the left when standing, but feels dizzy when turning to the left when lying down in bed. This is not vertebrobasilar ischaemia. Occasionally, however, one does not see a patient who has had a cervical manipulation and develops verte-brobasilar ischaemic attacks.

At angiography, it is relatively uncommon to find a cervical osteo-phyte distorting and compressing one of the vertebral arteries. Atheromatous changes in contrast are extremely common in the verte-brobasilar territory.

Cervical spondylosis usually causes nothing more than intermittent pain and some restriction of neck movement. It is unlikely to be the cause of the patient's symptoms in vertebrobasilar ischaemia. However, keeping the neck still by wearing a collar can be very helpful in reducing symptoms of postural or positional vertigo, because whatever the cause of the vestibular system damage, sudden change of position will tend to aggravate the symptoms.

Question 72.   What to do with whiplash?

Would you prefer a whiplash injury following a car accident resulting in a stiff, painful neck, but without abnormal X-ray or neurological deficit, to be treated with rest and a soft collar or anal-gesics and the encouragement of early mobilization, or a mixture of the two?

If there were, in addition, pain radiating to the shoulder or down one arm, would it make any difference to your management?

When a patient has just neck pain after a whiplash injury, the symptoms usually subside spontaneously after a few weeks. If the straight X-rays are normal, then the best course of management is to use a soft collar day and night, if tolerated, for the first 2 weeks together with some anal-gesics. Some patients seem to benefit more from anti-inflammatory analgesics than from paracetamol or co-proxamol. After 2 weeks, it is best to attempt to wean the patient off the collar but support with physio-therapy, if available, and continue the analgesics for a further few weeks.

Provided there is no compensation pending, then the pain tends to resolve. If there is compensation and the patient has been told that such an injury may well produce premature arthritis in the cervical spine, then discomfort is likely to persist.

When there is shoulder or arm pain, together with the neck pain, the concern is that one of the cervical nerve roots has been irritated or damaged.

If the patient's arm is examined carefully, one may find an area of weakness or sensory change confined to one of the nerve root territories, usually C5, C6 or C7. It is quite common to find depressed supinator and biceps reflex and brisk triceps response. The usual cause, however, is a prolapsed disc; the recommended treatment is to use a soft collar during the night and if necessary a firm collar during the day for 4–6 weeks. The patient will certainly need analgesics and may respond better to a combination with a muscle relaxant such as diazepam.

Patients are often in quite severe pain and, at times, there is a temptation to use steroids; often they are very beneficial as far as reducing pain is concerned. Other techniques including acupuncture or transcutaneous nerve stimulation may be tried.

Occasionally the pains do not settle, the neurological problems become more obvious and the patient may need to go on to have an MRI scan. This most efficiently confirms, or excludes, a significant underlying structural cause. It can be of great value in medico-legal cases.

Question 73.   'Not unless it's really necessary!' – cervical disc surgery

A woman solicitor aged 47 has had considerable trouble with her cervical spine. A surgeon has suggested that an operation might help, but does not push her. Her brother has had a laminectomy for lumbar disc problems. 'Would this be similar?' she asks. What kinds of operation are available?

Cervical disc surgery is never lightly undertaken as the surgical risks are much greater than those met in lumbar surgery. In lumbar surgery, significant paralysis is unlikely and, if it does occur, it will only be in one nerve root distribution. However, if something goes wrong with cervical surgery, then the spinal cord may be traumatized or infarcted and severe paralysis result. Fortunately, this is rare, but every year our medical defence societies have to pay out large sums for this complication of surgery. Also the beneficial effects of surgery are somewhat disappointing in the significant proportion of patients – even after what has been a technically good operation.

Long-term neurological problems are more common in the cervical spine than in the lumbar region, possibly because there is more movement in the cervical area. For example, if two vertebrae are fused in the neck, then within a few years there will be evidence of significant spondylosis at the disc spaces above and below the fusion.

The three main operative possibilities are:

1. Facetectomy – this is useful for decompressing vulnerable nerve roots from behind and can produce considerable pain relief and some return of function.
2. Laminectomy – this is an old-fashioned operation of taking the laminae off from behind to achieve decompression of the spinal cord. This is a big operation with the risk of infarcting the cord and not really suitable for the patient under discussion.

3. Cloward procedure – here the prolapsed disc is removed from in front (access is much easier than you might expect because the vertebral bodies are not far away from the front of the neck). After the disc has been removed, bony fragments extracted from the iliac crest are inserted to achieve a bony fusion. This is often a very successful operation and afterwards patients tend to complain more about the site of the bone removal from the iliac crest than about the neck!

In view of the fact that cervical surgery is potentially dangerous and a proportion of patients may be disappointed with the surgical result, you should never attempt to talk a patient into having surgery – especially if she is a solicitor! It really should be left to the patient who has been fully advised of the pros and cons of surgical treatment for her disc to ask for surgery. The vast majority of patients will settle on conservative management.

Question 74.   The when and why of back referral

A GP sees many cases of backache in the surgery. Most are simple and resolve more or less rapidly. How seriously should he or she consider the problem with regard to urgent referral if one of the following is present:

1. **An absent ankle jerk?**
2. **Unilateral sciatic pain sufficient to make work impossible?**
3. **Unilateral foot drop?**
4. **Bilateral sciatic discomfort not severe enough to make work impossible?**
5. **Paraesthesiae of the legs?**

The GP should arrange a full blood count, ESR, calcium and alkaline phosphatase. Lumbosacral X-rays are now rarely indicated. MRI scanning of the spine is free from ionizing radiation (important in this gonadal area) and is much more informative, showing discs and nerve roots as well as bony changes. Radiculography is now almost never necessary. An MRI scan showing no abnormality would encourage early mobilization whereas 2 weeks' bed rest would be advised in most cases of prolapsed disc.

The answers for points (1)–(5) are:

1. No need to refer unless there are other features.
2. It depends upon the family doctor's assessment. The patient should be genuine and failing to recover after 6 weeks, despite conservative measures such as bed rest and anti-inflammatory drugs before considering surgery.

3. Immediate investigation is advised although the cause may be something as simple as a lateral popliteal nerve lesion. A common scenario, unfortunately, is for the patient to be in agony with sciatica and then develop weakness on dorsiflexing one foot. The sciatica then decreases but the foot drop increases. By the time the pain has receded the nerve root has become infarcted and the recovery of the foot drop is likely to be poor.
4. This is urgent. Bilateral sciatic pain can indicate a central disc prolapse. It may result in pressure on the nerves of the sphincters. Any delay in treatment could result in incontinence and impotence. Some orthopaedic surgeons ask their neurosurgical colleagues to operate on such cases.
5. This is unlikely to be from a disc but could be caused by another centrally placed lesion. Refer to exclude other pathologies such as peripheral neuritis and Guillain–Barré syndrome.

Note: Neurologically speaking, traction is of little value in back pain except in keeping the patient tied down in bed!

Question 75.   Pain in the calves – normal pulses?

A man of 55 has pain in the calves when he walks which goes when he rests. To your surprise, you find that he has easily palpable foot pulses. What could be the explanation for this pain?

This patient is probably suffering from spinal claudication. The cause is usually a lumbar canal stenosis, and the cause of this is frequently multifactorial. Usually, there is a congenitally narrowed lumbar spine making it more vulnerable to degenerative changes which occur, such as multiple disc prolapses, osteophyte formation and hypertrophy of the posterior ligaments. Radiculography usually shows pinching of the column of contrast opposite the L5/S1, L4/L5 and the L3/L4 disc spaces.

The nerves are more greedy for blood than are the muscles. An increase in nerve blood flow is needed when exercising. The simplistic explanation for what occurs in spinal stenosis is that, with a narrowed canal, there is restriction on the necessary vasodilatation to supply the nerves' metabolic needs during exercising and pain results. Certainly such patients tend NOT to have pain come on so readily when they are cycling or going upstairs where the spine is flexed and the lumbar canal opens up a little and the chance of compression is less than when standing and walking.

So a patient who presents with claudication with normal foot pulses should perhaps be referred to a neurologist rather than a vascular surgeon.

Question 76.   Subacute combined – can you see it coming?

Can the symptoms of subacute combined degeneration of the cord precede:

- The anaemia of pernicious anaemia?
- The development of macrocytes?
- An abnormally low serum vitamin B$_{12}$?

Yes, yes and probably not. So keep an eye on the vitamin B$_{12}$ level in patients with dementia, spinal cord disease and peripheral neuropathy, even if there is no macrocytosis, as long as you can exclude other obvious causes and can justify this 'expensive' investigation to your thrifty haematologist.

Question 77.   Progressive spinal cord compression

A 46-year-old policeman complains of a 6-month progressive pain-less weakness of his right leg; he can no longer run, has had several trips and falls, one of which occurred recently while attempting to chase a criminal who thereby got away. His colleagues wonder whether 'he has lost his bottle'. Otherwise he has been very well. What is likely to be wrong and would a routine neurological appointment suffice?

- He may have spinal cord compression.
- Anyone with an undiagnosed progressive disability should be seen promptly.

With his history, it is important to check that he has had no past history of disc disease and sciatica, there have been no spinal injuries and he should be asked directly about whether he had had any symptoms in the other leg or any sphincter symptoms. You should ensure that his arms are normal, that he hasn't had any cranial nerve features or headache and you should enquire for any sensory change.

On examining him, you will probably find that both legs are weak, the reflexes may be brisk and the plantar responses extensor. Although there are no symptoms of sensory disturbance in many cases, you can demonstrate a sensory level in the trunk. The arms and cranial nerves are usually normal. You may be surprised sometimes that there is intention tremor in one hand with some nystagmus and a pale disc; it is not unknown for multiple sclerosis to present in this way and there is a subvariety where the patient demonstrates a progressive spastic para-paresis. There is also a familial variety of progressive spastic paraparesis and so the doctor should ask tactfully about other disability in the family.

Patients wiil usually need to be admitted to hospital for investigation which usually requires an MRI scan of the spine or, very occasionally these days, a myelogram. Very often at this age, the cause of the spinal cord compression is benign and an almost complete recovery can be expected if the lesion is removed. In older individuals, particularly men over 60 years, spinal deposits, particularly carcinoma of the prostate, need to be considered.

Infections

Question 78. Missable meningitis

A worried husband has called the doctor to see his normally healthy 32-year-old wife. She has had occasional migraine which never lasts for more than a day and intermittent sciatica. She has had a headache now for 3 days and it is getting worse. On examination, she is slightly pyrexial, no neck stiffness, but Kernig's sign is possibly positive on the side of the sciatica. What action should the doctor take?

Admit her to hospital urgently to exclude a meningitis.

The early stages of meningitis are not to be missed. If you have even thought of it, you should send the patient to hospital for assessment, observation and probable CSF examination.

It is not rare for a patient to have back pain or a positive Kernig's sign as prominent features of meningitis before neck stiffness is marked. Clearly, it is more difficult to be sure in this particular case with her past history of sciatica, but it is safer to assume that the positive Kernig's sign does, in fact, indicate a meningitis.

No one will ever criticize a family doctor for sending the patient into hospital with a ?meningitis – you won't be accused of crying wolf. It is well appreciated that many infectious diseases, such as 'flu, are accompanied by severe throbbing headaches without there being any significant clinical meningeal involvement, but I suspect that many such cases would show increased numbers of lymphocytes in their CSF but happily go on to spontaneous recovery.

It is probably not sensible to prescribe a broad-spectrum antibiotic and arrange to review the patient at home in 48 hours. If the antibiotic chosen proves to be ineffective and the patient goes on to develop more obvious features of meningitis, then the causative organism may be elusive. It is then necessary to treat the patient in the 'bacteriological dark' with a combination of powerful antibiotics.

If it could be a meningococcal infection, however, see Question 79.

Question 79.   Meningococcal meningitis – acute emergency!

An urban GP is encouraged to carry soluble penicillin in his bag lest he encounters a case of meningococcal meningitis. He sees little point in this as the patient would most probably be in hospital within half an hour. Is this view justified?

No. Even the smallest delay might be fatal.

Meningococcal meningitis is an awful illness. Treatment should be started the moment it is suspected. If the doctor diagnoses the condition correctly and gives penicillin, then a life might be saved. If the diagnosis is wrong and penicillin is given, little, if any, harm has been done.

Question 80.   Herpes simplex encephalitis

A man nearly dies as a result of an attack of herpes simplex encephalitis. He is left with considerable brain damage. Is there a type of person particularly at risk from this condition and should special precautions be taken if there was further exposure to herpes virus, for example, if one of the children had cold sores? What is the place of acyclovir in the treatment and prevention of herpes simplex encephalitis?

Herpes simplex virus may cause a devastating encephalitis involving primarily the temporal lobes. We are all exposed to herpes simplex. Only a tiny minority acquire the encephalitis – presumably due to an immunological defect, possibly a temporary one. They tend not to be chronic cold sore sufferers. The source of the infection is invariably obscure.

With such extensive involvement of the temporal lobes, there may be a major memory problem in those who survive. It is especially recent memory that is damaged, so that patients cannot retain any new information.

Acyclovir has been a major advance in the treatment of herpes virus infections. It protects some patients from going on to develop severe brain disease and acyclovir (or famciclovir, or valaciclovir) treatment is now instituted immediately the diagnosis is suspected. There is of course a theoretical risk that its use may preserve the lives of some individuals who would otherwise have died only to leave them with severe memory problems.

Sometimes the memory problems are so considerable that every moment it may seem to the patient that he has just woken up from a very long sleep. He may request his lunch 2 minutes after finishing a large meal; he might, when meeting his loved ones, whom he has seen only a few minutes before, greet them as though they have been separated from him for years. Nevertheless, for every case like this, perhaps kept alive by acyclovir, I suspect there will be tens of cases who will have minimal defects only. I would therefore use acyclovir in all but the moribund.

Clearly, one would want to spare such a patient from any further brain damage, but the chance of a further attack is remote. Although I have never known a case with a second attack of herpes simplex encephalitis, it is a theoretical risk and the family may be reassured by giving the patient some acyclovir orally and the child some acyclovir cream.

Question 81. Treating herpes zoster – is the expense justified?

A man aged 60 comes to the surgery with a recent eruption of herpes zoster lesions on his chest. A fairly mild case of shingles is diagnosed. Would you consider the use of oral and local acyclovir in such a case, bearing in mind the high cost of the treatment?

I think that if I was a GP, I would treat, with acyclovir, or famciclovir, or valaciclovir, virtually every case of herpes zoster I encountered in patients over the age of 60 and a significant proportion of those below 60, and all cases when the head or face was involved.

The greatest problem with herpes zoster is postherpetic neuralgia. Many patients are going to escape it, but some are going to be driven to desperation, even to suicide, by the chronic, awful pain. But which ones? There's the rub.

Not all severe postherpetic neuralgia occurs on the scalps and faces of people over 60. Occasionally postherpetic neuralgia can be severe in the young, in relatively 'insensitive' parts of the body and, sometimes, after relatively minimal skin lesions.

There is no effective protocol for the treatment of postherpetic neuralgia (see Question 89), and no proven one for its prevention.

The evidence suggests that, in a proportion of cases appropriate anti-viral medication, given in adequate doses, does seem to reduce the severity of postherpetic neuralgia. Until it is proved that it does not, I think I would continue to use it.

Visual problems and similar

Question 82. Homonymous hemianopia

As a result of a cerebrovascular accident, a man of 56 develops a homonymous hemianopia. He is most distressed because he has difficulty reading and watching television. His doctor reassures him that although the visual field defect may remain unaltered, his brain will probably accommodate and he will be able to enjoy both reading and viewing again. Is the doctor's optimism justified? Will the patient be allowed to drive again?

Possibly not. It is a sad observation that many field defects following stroke tend to be permanent. It is not necessary to be too pessimistic in the early days after a stroke if all that is found is a visual inattention on one side, because this often recovers. However, if there is still a homonymous field defect present in 2 weeks, it usually persists.

As far as enjoyment of reading and viewing is concerned, involvement of the central (macular) vision is critical. Indeed, macular vision is so important that the part of the visual cortex responsible for it has a dual blood supply from both the middle cerebral artery and the posterior cerebral artery on the ipsilateral side. Therefore, many patients who have had a stroke producing homonymous hemianopia will have some macular sparing, even if it is incomplete (Figure 1).

You can test for macular sparing quite simply by asking the patient to cover one eye and to fix on your pupil with the uncovered eye. You can then bring a target in from the blind half-field and if the patient can see it before it reaches the midline on the horizontal axis, then there is evidence of macular sparing and you can be reasonably optimistic that the patient will be able to watch television and to read, even though not with the previous speed. If the macular vision is split, then reading will be very laborious. With a left homonymous field defect, the patient will have difficulty finding the start of words and start of lines and, with a right homonymous field defect, difficulty finding the end of words and the end of lines. Patients can sometimes be helped by having a brightly coloured book mark which is placed at the beginning of each line or at the end of each line depending on the side of the hemianopia; when the eye meets the book mark, they then know they have reached the start or end of the line. Unfortunately, reading tends to remain very laborious and gives little pleasure to people with macular involvement.

For many patients of this age, a major frustration is not being able to drive. The Driving Licence Authority quite rightly will not consider it in patients with a homonymous hemianopia because of the risks involved in missing objects on the affected side. Patients with macular sparing may resent this restriction, because for most of the time they, like

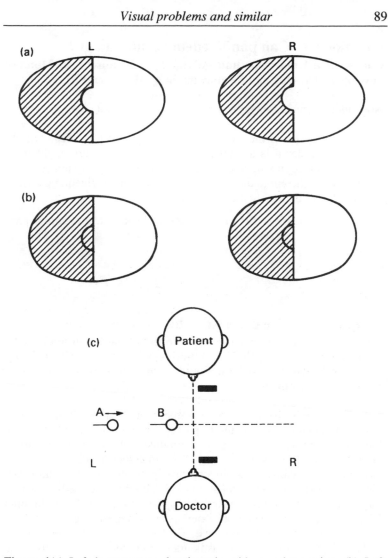

Figure 1(a) Left homonymous hemianopia with macular sparing. (b) Left homonymous hemianopia with macular involvement. Reading will be difficult, especially finding the beginning of lines and words. (c) Testing for macular involvement in a patient with a right homonymous hemianopia. If the patient can see the target at point B on the horizontal axis, before the midline is reached, then the macula is not involved.

everybody else, are very central field orientated. Those who cannot appreciate their problem may also have a visual association area lesion where there is inadequate appreciation of the field defect.

Question 83. Can papilloedema come and go?

Can papilloedema come and go rapidly – be absent on Monday, develop on Tuesday and be gone again by Wednesday?

No. Papilloedema might come on over a few hours but never resolves as quickly.

Headache is one of the most common complaints to be dealt with by a GP. Papilloedema is a vital physical sign and doctors ought to be competent at recognizing it. Dilating eye drops are usually unnecessary. It is usually sufficient to darken the room to obtain the fleeting glance of the disc that is all that should be required.

Note: Papilloedema is not always present in raised intracranial pressure!

Question 84. 'He can't keep his eyes open!'

A 64-year-old part-time drummer complains that he cannot keep his eyes open for any length of time and it is interfering with reading, watching television and he has had to give up driving. Can he be offered any treatment?

Yes. The two most likely causes are either that he has ocular myasthenia with an intermittent bilateral ptosis or that he has idiopathic blepharospasm. One can usually distinguish between them on simple clinical testing. In myasthenia, there is often associated diplopia and eye closure is invariably weak. In contrast, patients with blepharospasm appear just to be blinking a lot and keeping their eyes closed in a voluntary way. There is no weakness of eye closure and no diplopia. Blepharospasm is not a neurotic phenomenon in most cases, but it is one of the degenerative dystonic states.

The diagnosis of ocular myasthenia can be confirmed by giving an intravenous injection of edrophonium. If it is positive, further investigation to exclude a thymoma is required and the patient usually will respond better to steroid therapy on alternate days than to anticholinesterase drugs such as pyridostigmine alone.

Until quite recently, blepharospasm was more difficult to treat and various surgical procedures were recommended. Nowadays, it is possible to give very good symptomatic relief by injecting botulinum toxin into the orbicularis muscle. This usually gives relief for some months and then the injection can be repeated producing further relief. Patients are usually extremely grateful that their condition has been recognized and they can see again.

Question 85.   Is the optician incompetent?

A girl of 16 goes to the optician for a new pair of spectacles because her visual acuity is not as good as she would wish. Everybody in her family wears spectacles. After the examination, the optician says he cannot improve on her present state. Coincidentally, the next door neighbour, an elderly lady of 74, goes to the same optician and says that in spite of the spectacles he has given her, she cannot read or watch the television. Have both of them chosen a lousy optician? If not, what might be the explanation and is the explanation likely to be the same in the two cases? What should be done?

- The optician is likely to be competent.
- His findings imply that the visual problems are not due to a refractive error, but imply a medical cause.
- The cause is unlikely to be the same in the two age groups.
- The patients should be referred to an ophthalmologist promptly and if no ocular cause is found, referred on to a neurologist.

The ophthalmological causes will be quite different in the two groups. The 16-year-old girl might be found to have optic atrophy, possibly as a result of old inflammation or pressure but, in this age group, unlikely to be toxic. She may have a choroiditis from toxoplasmosis, or toxocariasis. She may have retinitis pigmentosa. She is not likely to have Leber's optic atrophy which is an X-linked disorder and is therefore more likely in teenage boys.

The elderly woman is most likely to have cataracts, senile macular degeneration, glaucoma or a diabetic or hypertensive retinopathy.

Neurologically, the concern in the two patients is about the possibility of a compressive lesion producing the visual failure. Again the causes are different in the two age groups. In the teenage girl, there is a possibility that she might have optic nerve glioma or a mass in the pituitary region, perhaps a craniopharyngioma. Optic neuritis is another common possibility, even at this age. It should always be remembered that it is not uncommon for teenage girls to complain of visual impairment and no organic cause can be found. With encouragement and observation, the visual problem sometimes corrects itself.

In the elderly patient, tumours in the pituitary region are quite common, including primary pituitary adenomas, metastases, aneurysm and meningiomas. Non-compressive causes would include optic atrophy from vitamin B_{12} deficiency, syphilis or diabetes and also vascular lesions involving the optic nerve. Hemisphere lesions usually produce a homonymous hemianopia and do not commonly present an uncorrectable problem with visual acuity.

The neurological investigation of these patients would include a skull X-ray which might show an abnormal pituitary fossa with suprasellar calcification; the optic foramina might be enlarged. Visual evoked responses would be expected to be abnormal. If they were normal in the teenage girl, then one would suspect a non-organic cause for the visual symptoms. The blood tests should include assessment of the vitamin B_{12} and blood sugar. Syphilis serology is particularly necessary in the elderly woman whose husband might have brought back the treponeme as one of his medals from the Second World War. High resolution CT or MRI scanning of the orbital pituitary regions is necessary and, if normal, a compressive cause for the visual failure can be virtually excluded. CSF examination may be necessary in the teenage girl to exclude demyelination and in the old lady to look for neoplastic cells, as she may have a malignant infiltration of her basal meninges.

Poor visual acuity which cannot be corrected by the optician is an important finding and should never be ignored.

Question 86. Visual field defect and the lorry driver

A lorry driver aged 35 complains of disturbing transient episodes from which he loses half of his visual field for 20 minutes. He has no headache afterwards. He has been told by a previous doctor that these attacks are just migraine. What would you tell him? Would you advise further investigations?

'... if such attacks are liable to develop suddenly and without any prodromal signs, restriction of driving should be considered.'
Medical Aspects of Fitness to Drive (1985), p 57.

It is only too easy to dismiss all transient visual disturbances as migraine. The patient should be told that these attacks are not to be ignored, not only because of their medical implications but also as far as his job is concerned. He must be informed that further assessment is required and a neurological referral arranged.

In migraine, there is usually a degree of warning. Often visual disturbance – zig-zags, stars, etc. – present before there is actual loss of visual field. Sometimes there is no subsequent headache, just a feeling of being unwell. If the lorry driver were at other times to have typical migraine with eye signs, hemisensory changes, hemicranial headache and nausea or vomiting, this would make it even more likely that the isolated attacks of visual disturbance were migrainous in origin. But the neurologist would certainly want to check for any permanent visual field defect.

In the vast majority of cases, the history and clinical examination is all that is required, but in a minority, investigations are advised. The development of anaemia is sometimes the cause for an exacerbation of the patient's migraine and certainly full blood count, ESR and platelet count should be performed. The blood sugar should be checked and, in a very small minority of patients, CT scanning and possibly CSF examination would be indicated.

It should be made very clear to the patient that there are two aspects of his problem. First, the medical control of his attacks and, secondly, how the problem influences, not only his professional driving licence, but also his ability to drive socially. First, he should be advised to avoid the common things which aggravate migraine, such as going without sleep and going for long periods without food. Perhaps he has noticed these attacks are more likely to come on after he has had coffee, cheese or chocolate and he may have noticed that even small amounts of alcohol trigger an attack, not necessarily the same day, but the day after.

There is a risk that in one of the attacks, the visual disturbance may not be temporary and a permanent visual field defect might result. For this reason, he should stop smoking and possibly take an aspirin a day as an antiplatelet gesture. The patient might also benefit from a migraine prophylactic such as low dose clonidine or propranolol. If the lorry driver is female, she should stop the oral contraceptive pill.

Driving advice

You should ensure from the outset that the patient realizes that you are trying to help, that you are acting as his medical adviser and that you are not the spy of the Driving Licence Authority. You should emphasize that you are looking for grounds to allow him to continue to drive, rather than looking for an excuse to ban him from driving.

Certainly, he should be told that he should stop driving immediately at the first sign of one of the migraine attacks coming on. This might be easier for a lorry driver than for drivers of public service vehicles. A taxi driver, for example, is in a way more of a worry, because he might be driving a fare down the M4 at speed in order to catch an aeroplane. He is unlikely to pull over to the hard shoulder on the motorway and wait for his vision to recover.

Often, the visual disturbance isn't the main neurological problem which occurs in migraine episodes; patients often complain much more about the lack of concentration which continues for some hours. They often describe this as if the mind has been scrambled and clearly driving under these circumstances is not to be advised.

If the patient makes a good response to changes in his lifestyle and to migraine prophylactic agents, such that he gets only very infrequent attacks and these are invariably accompanied by some predictable and satisfactory warning, then he probably does not constitute a driving hazard. The patient who has attacks of sudden visual loss may well need to be barred from driving, albeit temporarily.

Finally, when advising such a patient, the doctor should ask how he or she would stand if something were to go wrong and the patient did have an accident. The doctor would be open to criticism, not only from the patient and his family, but also the possible victims of any collision. If in any doubt at all, you must persuade the patient to consult the Driving Licence Authority.

Question 87. Visual obscuration on standing – a significant symptom

A man aged 47 who is a heavy smoker says that sometimes, when he stands up, his vision goes dull for a second or two. He adds that he has recently developed some headache, but has previously been well with a blood pressure of 140/80. Need anything be done about this?

Yes. He should be referred urgently. This symptom almost certainly indicates a serious pathology.

Transient visual disturbances in patients with headache are usually labelled as migraine. Clearly this is not the case with this particular patient. Visual symptoms with migraine are not usually posturally related and they nearly always last for more than just a few seconds.

The patient complains of visual obscuration on standing. This implies an underperfusion of the retina or occipital lobes with the transient postural fall in blood pressure. This is most commonly due to raised intracranial pressure or to severe arterial disease.

In patients with recent onset of headache, visual obscuration on standing is due to papilloedema and possible cerebral tumour until proved otherwise. Urgent referral is suggested. In a smoker aged 47, by far the most common type of cerebral tumour would be a cerebral metastasis from a carcinoma of the bronchus, but sometimes we are pleasantly surprised.

In a more elderly patient with possibly some other hint of vascular disease, the possibility of significant stenosis of the carotid, retinal or vertebral arteries should be questioned. In this case, the patients do not typically have a related headache.

These arteriopaths usually have evidence of bruits in the neck; they also require urgent referral. This type of symptom may occasionally occur in cranial arteritis, but this man is too young for this disease.

Patients with autonomic failure, e.g. resulting from diabetes, may have substantial drops in blood pressure when upright. They tend not to lose vision immediately on standing, but vision tends to fade as the blood pressure starts to fall as a result of remaining in the upright position.

Question 88. Diplopia and squint – neurologist or ophthalmologist?

A woman aged 47 suddenly develops diplopia. She feels otherwise very well. Would you suggest she be referred to an optician, ophthalmologist or a neurologist? What referral would you suggest for her 5-year-old grand-daughter who has recently developed a squint?

Granny should see the neurologist. Grand-daughter should see an ophthalmologist.

Some visual problems are referred appropriately to the optician in the first instance. Certainly refer a patient with sudden onset diplopia which developed as a direct result of bifocal spectacles recently prescribed. This is not uncommon! It is exceptional for opticians to suggest a neurological opinion; possibly it goes against the normal referral channel.

Most cases are referred to the ophthalmologist who then sends the vast majority to the neurologist for assessment. It would be appropriate, therefore, for the GP to send most cases of diplopia directly to the neurological department.

Diplopia, by its very nature, is nearly always of sudden onset. It is only rarely due to an intraocular cause, a dislocated lens for example. Quite frequently, it is caused by a third, fourth or sixth nerve lesion on one side which has resulted from injury or vascular disease (hypertension, diabetes, syphilis). It may be a symptom of an intracranial space-occupying lesion. Other causes of double vision are multiple sclerosis and myasthenia gravis. Some patients develop diplopia when they decompensate for a longstanding squint – often occurring at the time of intercurrent illness or surgical operation.

In the case of the 5-year-old grand-daughter, referral to the optician is equally inappropriate. In most cases, a direct referral to the ophthalmologist should be made. An isolated squint in a child is very rarely due to neurological disease.

If, however, other features such as diplopia (most children with a squint do NOT complain of diplopia), headache, vomiting, ataxia or abnormal clumsiness have developed, then an urgent neurological referral should be made. The possible diagnosis in this case? A posterior fossa tumour. The most common solid tumours in children are found in the posterior fossa.

As medicine becomes more and more complex, it is of prime importance for the family doctor to point the patient in the right direction. In countries where multi-speciality clinics have in the main replaced the family doctor, patients can flounder in a very expensive, if not critically delayed, fashion before arriving at the right doorstep.

Pain problems

Question 89. The problem of postherpetic neuralgia

Is there an accepted protocol to use in the treatment of distressing postherpetic neuralgia of the face which has not responded to mild analgesics alone?

No. The first division of the trigeminal nerve is frequently involved with herpes zoster eruption whereas the second and third divisions are usually the territory of the herpes simplex virus. Postherpetic neuralgia on the face is therefore nearly always in the first division. Trigeminal neuralgia is more common in the second and third divisions.

Established postherpetic neuralgia is a misery. It is very resistant to treatment, particularly in the elderly. With elderly patients, after a while, it is almost as if they have nothing else to live for but their pain. It becomes more dominating and they develop chronic pain behaviour. Many become severely depressed and even suicidal.

Simple analgesics are usually useless on their own. A more powerful analgesic such as co-proxamol, co-dydramol or codeine, often used in combination with a simple analgesic and caffeine, nearly always has to be resorted to. Patients should not be given more powerful opiates unless the situation is desperate, because the risk of addiction is high.

Patients nearly always need an antidepressant and sometimes benefit from chlorpromazine and/or carbamazepine in addition.

Unfortunately, nerve section and nerve injections and blocks are of no use because the cause of the pain is central in patients with established postherpetic neuralgia. Local treatment to the painful area other than with bland ointments is usually unpopular and transcutaneous nerve stimulation and acupuncture can actually make the pain worse.

The hope is that active treatment of herpes zoster eruptions in the acute phase with a combination of local acyclovir plus acyclovir by mouth or by injection will reduce the chance of postherpetic neuralgia and possibly its severity.

Also in the early phases analgesics should be used enthusiastically in an attempt to prevent the pain becoming a habit.

Paradoxically, I am less concerned about trying to prevent postherpetic neuralgia in the first division of the trigeminal nerve than elsewhere. Most patients will be referred promptly to an ophthalmologist because of concern about the preservation of sight and prompt treatment is usually instituted. However, little eruptions of shingles on the trunk may not be treated very enthusiastically and may result in crippling postherpetic pain.

Question 90.   Carpal tunnel syndrome – is surgery really necessary?

A 25-year-old mother complains of pain and tingling in one hand. The GP thinks this is due to a carpal tunnel syndrome. Should he send the patient directly to a surgeon?

No. Although carpal tunnel syndrome is quite a likely diagnosis, there are a number of other important possibilities. I frequently get asked to see patients whose hand symptoms have failed to respond to carpal tunnel decompression and these could have been spared surgery.

First, determine that the sensory disturbances are confined to the territory of the median nerve and not overlapping into the ulnar nerve territory. Ask whether the symptoms come on with the typical pattern of waking her at night and then coming on with knitting, peeling vegetables etc.? Is she pregnant? Is she on the oral contraceptive pill? Are there any signs of hypothyroidism? Is she diabetic? Is she overweight?

On examining the arms, you should ensure that any muscle wasting is confined to the thenar eminence, that there is no evidence of any proximal weakness or weakness in the small muscles of the hands, innervated by the ulnar nerve. The reflexes should be normal. The sensory disturbances should be confined to the territory of the median nerve. Check that the patient has no evidence of any less prominent problems on the other side, or any sensory disturbance in the feet (to suggest a peripheral neuropathy).

Simple investigations should include a full blood count, ESR, blood sugar and a TSH. If there is any hint of arthritis, check the rheumatoid factors. EMG and nerve conduction studies would need to be performed before the patient had carpal tunnel decompression.

The vast majority of patients can be managed without any surgical intervention. Correcting any metabolic problem may suffice; getting the patient to lose weight, using a cock-up splint to wear at night and corticosteroid injection into the carpal tunnel might all be tried.

To ensure a good operative result, it is necessary to demonstrate a delay in electrical conduction in the median nerve across the carpal ligament.

Question 91. Unremitting faceache

A 41-year-old housewife with a demanding young family and a difficult husband consults you about severe pain in her face. She has already been to the dentist and had some teeth removed – to no avail. What are the likely causes? How should one proceed?

The likely causes of the facial pain at this age are:

● Toothache.
● Sinusitis.
● Trigeminal neuralgia.
● Atypical facial pain.
● A migraine variant.

You should take a more detailed history and examine her face. What is the character of the pain? What are the associated features? Is there any sinus tenderness? Do the remaining teeth look healthy? Is the nose blocked? Is there much catarrh? Are there any trigger spots where the lightest touch triggers off the painful spasm? Is there any sensory loss on the face? Are the corneal reflexes normal? Is the patient depressed?

Toothache of course is a very common cause of facial pain at this age, but usually when the offending tooth has been removed, the pain subsides. However, it is quite common for the patient to make the wrong self-diagnosis and to insist that the dentist removes several teeth before accepting that another cause must be responsible.

Sinusitis is usually quite easy to diagnose or to exclude and one would be in difficulties trying to defend this diagnosis if a patient had a perfectly clear nose with no facial tenderness. If these features are present, then prompt antibiotic treatment is recommended. If the pain fails to clear up satisfactorily, sinus X-rays should be recommended.

Trigeminal neuralgia can occur in young people although more typically it is found in the elderly. If it does occur in the young, you should think of a possible underlying cause such as demyelination. The character of the pain is absolutely typical with sudden, shooting spasms of pain lasting just a few seconds, often triggered by touch, talking, cleaning the teeth, eating, with very many spasms occurring during the day. In between the spasms, there may be a slight background 'awareness' but there is no actual pain. Trigeminal sensation should be perfectly normal.

If there is trigeminal sensory loss, one should consider an infiltrative lesion of the trigeminal nerve. Further investigation via the neurological department is recommended. In other parts of the world where nasopharyngeal carcinomas are much more common than in the UK, facial pain and sensory loss are much more likely to be due to a sinister underlying cause.

The treatment of trigeminal neuralgia is often very gratifying and the patient should be gradually introduced to carbamazepine, initially 50 mg at night increasing by 50 mg every day or two until the patient has pain relief. It you put a patient straight on to 100 mg carbamazepine three times a day, she may feel rotten and then refuse to take it subsequently. If carbamazepine alone fails to work, phenytoin could be added; patients usually go into remission after a few days on treatment and when free of pain for a period of a few weeks, the treatment can be gradually reduced and then reintroduced when there is a relapse. If the pain becomes too severe to be controlled by medication, then thermocoagulation of the trigeminal nerve can be tried. This is now preferable to injecting the nerve with alcohol.

Nagging unilateral facial pain with no abnormal signs but a hint that the patient might be depressed is sometimes labelled atypical facial pain. The patients most often respond to an antidepressant, but they rarely accept this without investigation and unfortunately neurological referral is probably necessary!

Urinary difficulty

Question 92.   Stress incontinence – don't forget your neurology!

A woman aged 57, otherwise well, has stress incontinence. On examination the doctor finds that she has a moderate degree of anterior vaginal wall descent. Are there any factors in the history which might make the opinion of the neurologist more pertinent than that of a gynaecologist?

Stress incontinence is often mechanical and a gynaecological opinion may well be appropriate.

However, a minority may have symptoms which clearly indicate that there is more to it than a simple urethrocele.

Does the patient have any symptoms to suggest that there may be a local defect of sensation? She should be asked about the presence of perineal numbness. Can she feel herself passing urine? Can she feel herself wiping herself and, when she sits on a cold plastic lavatory seat, can she feel that it is cold? Does she have normal vaginal sensation? Does she sometimes leak without knowing it?

Is there any difficulty initiating micturition even when the bladder is full? If the woman has hesitancy, it is often worth looking further. In contrast, the symptom or urgency is not very helpful. Anyone who has lost confidence in the bladder will have diurnal urgency and frequency.

Nocturnal incontinence is very much against a simple, local mechanical cause and should point to there being an underlying neurological disturbance as well.

If the woman had had fairly substantial perineal injuries during childbirth, then anal sphincter control may be unsatisfactory. However, difficulty with anal sensation and control clearly points to the problem being more than a prolapse. Can she distinguish flatus from faeces? Is there any faecal incontinence? Can she feel the toilet paper?

Even though the patient may say that she is otherwise perfectly well, it is worth checking for the neurological conditions that can cause difficulty with bladder control outlined in Question 93.

Question 93.   Unsuccessful prostatectomy

A man aged 52 has a prostatectomy for difficulty in passing urine. He is no better afterwards. Comment?

This is quite a common neurological referral. However, the patients are usually more elderly than this man, when it has been assumed that the prostate was responsible on fairly sound statistical if not clinical grounds. In a 52 year old, the chance of a significant prostatic hypertrophy is low and that of an alternative explanation is high.

First, the prostatectomy itself may have been unsatisfactory, so who did it? The medicolegal development in the UK is not sufficiently advanced to prevent the generalist from performing transurethral resection of the prostate and unfortunately some surgical results are a little disappointing.

However, the chances are that there was a neurological component to the patient's urinary symptoms and that just removing the prostate was not appropriate. In some cases, prostatectomy actually makes things much worse and the patients become incontinent.

The neurological conditions that can cause difficulty with bladder control are numerous:

- Spinal cord disease, including multiple sclerosis and compressive lesions.
- Severe lumbar canal stenosis and spondylosis pressing on the sacral nerve roots.
- Autonomic neuropathy, e.g. in diabetes.
- Dementia.
- Frontal lobe lesions.

So before you refer any patient for a prostatic opinion, ask:

- Has there been any past history of neurological disease?
- Is the patient well preserved mentally?
- Are there any difficulties with control of the anal sphincter? – if there are then clearly it is more than just a prostatic problem.
- Does the patient have any significant backache or sciatica?
- Is there any weakness of the legs or difficulty walking?
- Is there any sensory disturbance in the legs or on the buttocks and perineum?

If any one of these features is present, then perhaps the patient should be referred to a neurologist rather than urologist.

Miscellaneous

Question 94.   The tippler with painful feet

An overweight 55-year-old shopkeeper complains of a painful numbness of both feet. He is known to drink heavily. Can it safely be assumed that this is alcohol related and he just be given B vitamins?

No. If he is overweight and well fed, an alcoholic peripheral neuropathy is somewhat less likely than in the heavier drinker who neglects his diet.

The chances are that this man has a peripheral neuropathy. There are more causes of peripheral neuropathy than almost any other clinical presentation in neurology. In the UK, the two most common are due to diabetes which is often pain-free, but occasionally painful, and to alcohol abuse which is frequently accompanied by burning discomfort.

On examining the patient you may find that there is some early sensory disturbance he has been unaware of in the finger tips with a lack of appreciation of cotton wool and pinpick stimulation in the periphery, becoming more normal as the stimuli spread proximally. The peripheral reflexes may be reduced.

Investigation would be to exclude an underlying neoplasm particularly of the lung or kidney. A glucose tolerance curve is advised, vitamin B_{12} level should be estimated and serum protein electrophoresis performed in addition to a full blood count and ESR. At the neurological department, the patient should have nerve conduction studies carried out to distinguish between an axonal and myelin sheath neuropathy. Lumbar puncture is usually required to examine the CSF protein and electrophoretic pattern.

If it transpires that alcohol is the cause of his neuropathy, then stopping alcohol and giving high doses of B vitamins would produce a fairly prompt reduction of his pain and a slightly slower recovery in his peripheral sensory loss.

Question 95.   Neurological AIDS

A gay local travel agent has developed a peripheral sensory distance. He thinks he has AIDS. Can it present in this way?

Yes. As far as AIDS is concerned, this individual is at high risk. First he is homosexual and secondly he works as a travel agent and presumably the number of contacts he has, both in this country and overseas, particularly perhaps in the USA, would be greater than average.

Neurological problems in AIDS are legion. Some of my neurological colleagues think that AIDS is a neurological disease. Patients suffer not only the ravages of opportunistic infection, but also from tumours. In some American neurosurgical centres now, AIDS cases account for the majority of neurosurgical biopsies. Previous disastrous projections have, fortunately, not proved entirely accurate but it is still currently estimated that by the year 2000, I could be admitting as many as 5 AIDS patients per week to my neurological beds. Peripheral nerve problems are quite common, not just peripheral neuropathy, but also mononeuritis or a mononeuritis multiplex (a number of discrete peripheral nerve lesions). Spinal cord lesions also occur (myelitis). The patient may have meningitis or brain stem lesions or hemisphere problems including multiple cerebral abscesses.

You should tell the patient that there are many causes of peripheral neuropathy other than AIDS and that he needs neurological referral and investigation. Clearly he needs counselling before he has his HIV test and his consent must be obtained. Most patients who present in this way with this worry will usually agree to having the test performed.

Question 96. Writer's cramp

A 43-year-old building surveyor complains of difficulty writing. He develops pain and stiffness in his hand and forearm when he attempts to do so. What is the likely cause? What can be done about it?

- The likely cause is writer's cramp.
- Treatments include big pens, biofeedback and botulinum toxin!

The differential diagnosis here includes writer's cramp, parkinsonism, a pyramidal lesion and an ulnar nerve lesion. These four can usually be distinguished on clinical examination.

Typically, patients with writer's cramp have no abnormality on clinical examination until they are asked to write. The pen is then held very stiffly, writing is very laborious, tremulous with extreme tightness of the forearm muscles and, after a line or two, the patient has to give up. Invariably, the patient's occupation involves a lot of handwriting and it was felt for many years that this was a neurotic condition and there were possibly deep underlying psychological reasons for the patient not wishing to be able to write and thereby avoiding some conflict of interests at work.

Nowadays, writer's cramp is thought to be a focal dystonia with a defect in the complex reflex arc that is involved in the complicated function of writing. Often other fine movements like knitting, sewing or handiwork are unaffected.

Drug therapy is of little use. Psychiatric referral is almost never indicated. If the patient is reasonably ambidextrous, he can be taught to write with the other hand but there are numerous examples of patients going on to develop writer's cramp in the non-dominant hand as well! Various biofeedback techniques have been tried where surface EMG electrode helps record muscle action potentials which are then played on a loud speaker which the patient can hear. He then attempts to relax the affected muscles and thereby achieves a more satisfactory style of writing. Although these techniques may prove to be of temporary benefit in the long term, I have not found them to be very valuable. What can help some patients is to get them to use a fat, big pen, the ink of which flows smoothly and for the patient to be taught to hold the pen very lightly and to learn to write with the proximal arm and shoulder muscles rather than with the muscles of the hand and forearm. Injection of botulinum toxin has been tried with variable success.

Other patients respond better by using alternative methods of getting their thoughts onto paper. They could use a dictaphone and then would only need to sign their name. Sometimes, this is not possible and some patients have to find alternative employment. Hopefully, our building surveyor would be able to cope with a dictaphone and a good secretary. The patient is often helped considerably by your reassuring him that he has not got a neurotic condition.

Question 97.   Neurologist or paediatrician?

Below what age would you consider it reasonable for a patient with an apparent neurological problem to be referred in the first event to a paediatrician rather than to a neurologist?

Ideally, children with neurological problems should be seen by a paediatric neurologist. Neurological services are inadequate and badly distributed throughout the country. Paediatric neurologists are very sparsely distributed although ideally each region should have at least one.

Relatively few GPs are going to have direct access to a paediatric neurologist. The Royal College of Physicians recognizes that consultant neurologists might be expected to advise on children. They are now required to have some paediatric input during their general professional or higher specialist training in neurology.

Children under five should be referred directly to a paediatrician.

Over 5 years of age, most of the neurological problems will be familiar to an adult neurologist and you can take your choice depending on local availability and personalities. With some advantage, the management of a difficult neurological case of a child could be shared between a paediatrician and a neurologist.

Teenagers who present with neurological problems should probably be referred directly to an adult neurologist.

Question 98.   How reliable are CT scans?

How fallible are CT brain scans? Are there any lesions more likely to be missed than others?

For the anxious or hypochondriacal patient who is worried that he has a brain tumour, the CT scan should be regarded as infallible. Modern 'state of the art' scanners show intracranial detail that would have been thought impossible 15 years ago. It often helps reassure the patient if they are shown the scan and smaller details, such as the ocular lens, are demonstrated to show the power of the machine!

However, some lesions can be missed. The three important categories are cerebral infarcts, small lesions close to the bone and posterior fossa lesions. In essence, the CT scan is showing you a density picture. When infarcts are isodense with normal brain, they do not show. Lesions which are close to bone may be missed because bone is so extremely dense compared with soft tissue. The scan is prone to movement artefact, particularly in the posterior fossa where linear streaking may be sufficient to obscure an underlying small lesion.

The magnetic resonance scan is better than CT brain scanning in all three of the above problem areas. However, access to MRI scanners in the UK is still poor. It is sad that in the country where the scanners were invented and developed, clinical installations are far fewer than in other 'advanced' countries. If it is not possible to obtain an MRI scan in a patient about whom you are worried who has a normal CT brain scan in the early phase of his illness, then the advice is to wait and, if the symptoms persist, repeat the CT brain scan after a month or so. In many cases who have an underlying tumour, the abnormality will be demonstrated. In patients who have a significant hemiparesis of sudden onset with a normal CT scan, there can be reasonable confidence that the cause was a cerebral infarct.

Some of my neurological colleagues feel that the only interesting neurology nowadays is when the CT scan is normal!

Question 99.   Neurology, driving and the law

Advising the patient to stop driving and notifying the Driving Licence Authority of his condition seems a common occurrence in a number of neurological conditions. Could you please give a broad outline on how this is assessed in cases of epilepsy and other neurological problems?

It is necessary to consider two groups:

- Group 1: ordinary driving licence holders, which also includes those whose work requires long hours of driving, e.g. commercial representatives.
- Group 2: vocational driving licence holders who may be (1) Large Goods Vehicle (LGV) licence holders or (2) Passenger Carrying Vehicle (PCV) licence holders. These include minibus, taxi, ambulance and police drivers, some of whom may need to meet medical standards set by organizations other than the Driving Licence Authority.

A number of conditions, e.g. epilepsy, heart attack, diabetes, do require the driver to notify the Driving Licence Authority. The doctor should make it clear to the patient that he, or she, has such a condition and that it should be notified. It is the patient's responsibility to make that notification to the Driving Licence Authority. Any other action taken by the doctor is a breach of confidence and should only be undertaken in the most exceptional of circumstances. Certain guidelines have been laid down by the General Medical Council and advice from a medical defence society should be sought.

Epilepsy
For the purpose of driving a motor vehicle, epilepsy includes both major and minor seizures. A momentary lapse of consciousness on a motorway could have as devastating a result as a major seizure.

As soon as anybody has any kind of epileptic attack, whether awake or asleep, they should immediately stop driving and notify the Driving Licence Authority.

A Group 2 licence (LGV/PSV) may only be considered if the applicant has been free of any epileptic attack for 10 years, off treatment for 10 years and in whom there is no continuing liability to epilepsy, e.g. no structural intracranial lesion.

It is probably easier to say which person with epilepsy CAN drive. A private motorist with epilepsy can drive if:

- He has had no attack of any kind for 1 year.
- He has had attacks only whilst asleep, but never when awake, for a period of observation of 3 years, i.e. he has been proved to have 'sleep epilepsy'.
- His driving is not a source of danger to the public.

The licence given will be of a fixed period of from 1 to 3 years. If, at any time, the person has any kind of fit (except sleep epilepsy – the second category above) then he will have to stop driving until 1 year has passed without any manifestation of epilepsy.

In the case of a private motorist having a single fit, he should stop driving straight away and notify the Driving Licence Authority immediately. Usually a 12-month restriction will be imposed. Such patients should, of course, be fully and appropriately investigated.

If a professional driver has a fit he will lose his licence for 10 years. If he has a 'blackout of unknown cause' then he could also lose his licence for a prolonged period depending upon the decision of the Driving Licence Authority. Some professional drivers may be barred from any further participation in their occupation by their own licensing authority.

If a person who suffers from epilepsy wishes to come off his anticonvulsant therapy he must not drive whilst the medication is being withdrawn and for 6 months thereafter. If the person does have a fit in that time he does, unfortunately, lose his licence until 1 year free of fits has passed. For this reason, many people are reluctant to come off therapy once their fits are controlled.

Blackouts
These come under the general requirement to notify the Driving Licence Authority of 'sudden attacks of disabling giddiness or fainting' that could occur during driving.

It is not just unconsciousness from epilepsy that can put the driver off the road. Syncopal attacks for transient cerebral anoxia, as might happen with a cardiac arrhythmia, for example, should also be notified to the Driving Licence Authority.

Notifications should also be made in cases of sudden unconsciousness of an unknown cause. In the case of a private motorist, this will probably mean that driving will not be allowed for 1 year. In the case of the professional drivers, it might well mean a 5-year ban on their carrying on with their occupation.

Transient ischaemic attacks and stroke
Following a TIA, or very mild stroke, the Driving Licence Authority should be informed and the patient should not drive, socially, for at least a month. Patients having multiple TIAs should be stopped for longer, until satisfactory control of symptoms is achieved. A professional driver needing a Group 2 licence will probably be stopped for much longer and may not be allowed to resume his occupation. Many doctors forget to tell their patient to notify the Driving Licence Authority, particularly with the more minor episodes.

After a moderate stroke, driving may not be advisable for 6 months. At the end of that time an assessment of fitness to drive is carried out. Arrangements for this can be made at driving schools such as the British School of Motoring (BSM). Depending on the degree and nature of the residual disability, the licence is either restored or withdrawn for a further period. A person might, for example, be able to drive with some loss of power in a limb if adjustment is made to the car controls. He would not, however, be allowed to do so if he had developed such a condition as homonymous hemianopia or impairment of comprehension.

Note: These are but a few of the neurological reasons for notifying the Driving Licence Authority. Many other conditions that might affect the ability to drive also require notification: Menière's disease, established multiple sclerosis, dementia, Parkinson's disease, narcolepsy and motor neurone disease. In many such cases, however, the patient will be allowed to continue to drive unless, or until such a time as, the condition makes him a hazard to others. After a substantial head injury or craniotomy, the Driving Licence Authority will normally require a 12-month period of observation before driving is allowed again.

The situation regarding driving with cerebral tumours is particularly complex and a neurological opinion should be sought. Even more difficult is the patient who, whilst superficially appearing to be normal, is known to be in the early stages of dementia. In such a case a specialist opinion could be of great value.

For further information request a copy of *At a Glance Guide to Current Medical Standards of Fitness to Drive* from the Driving Licence Authority or *Medical Aspects of Fitness to Drive*, 1995.

Question 100. Urgent or non-urgent?

You have a long waiting list for appointments. What category of patient would you happily see urgently? Be most unhappy to do so?

- I would happily see anyone you are worried about.
- I would be unhappy to see someone who clearly does not have a neurological problem, but an anxiety state or psychosis.

It is somewhat difficult to be dogmatic and any list offered is bound to have some omissions. With these caveats, the following lists are suggested.

Symptoms requiring urgent neurological referral
Some of the following problems may require urgent admission rather than an urgent outpatient appointment.

1. Headache: (a) Patients with a sudden onset of headache which might be due to a subarachnoid haemorrhage or meningitis. Remember that patients with meningitis do not necessarily have neck stiffness. Admit.
    (b) Headaches of recent onset that are worse in the morning and increased by straining and coughing are particularly worrying. Patients with these features are suggestive of raised intracranial pressure especially when accompanied by focal neurological

symptoms. Do not be put off by the absence of papilloedema or your ability to detect it. Some patients with a raised intracranial pressure never develop papilloedema.

(c) Elderly patients with scalp tenderness where cranial arteritis is a possibility.

(d) Children with headaches and unsteadiness. Posterior fossa tumours are the most common childhood tumour (excluding the leukaemias, of course). Children often make little of their headaches, so don't expect a description typical of raised intracranial pressure. They rarely complain abut being unsteady.

2. Spinal cord compression – patients with symptoms suggestive of spinal cord compression, particularly if there are any urinary difficulties. If there is more than 24 hours delay in treating urinary difficulties due to spinal cord or cauda equina compression, adequate sphincter control may never be restored and male patients are usually rendered impotent. Admit.

3. Patients with *progressive neurological symptoms and signs*. If there is any disturbance of consciousness or alertness, they should be admitted.

4. Patients with transient ischaemic attacks or attacks of monocular blindness.

5. Troublesome epilepsy – more than two fits in succession and ? in early status. Admit.

Worrying symptoms which are uncommonly due to severe disease
Urgent referral of the following symptoms is not usually required and a routine appointment should suffice.

- Attacks of sudden vertigo without any brain stem signs such as diplopia, facial numbness or dysarthria.
- Longstanding headache.
- Back pain and sciatica.
- Postviral syndrome.
- Isolated convulsion.

Useful addresses

Age Concern
England: 60 Pitcairn Road, Mitcham, Surrey, CR4 3LL
Wales: 1 Park Grove, Cardiff, CF1 3BJ
Scotland: 33 Castle Street, Edinburgh, EH2 3DN
Northern Ireland: 128 Great Victoria Street, Belfast, BT2 7BG

Alcoholics Anonymous
General Service Office Great Britain, PO Box 1, Stonebow House, York
(Tel: 01904 644026)
For your nearest branch, see local telephone directory

Alzheimer Disease Society
Head Office, Bank Buildings, Fulham Broadway, London, SW6 1EP
(Tel: 0171 381 3177)

Association of Carers
1st Floor, 21/23 New Road, Chatham, Kent, ME4 4QJ (Tel: 01634
813981)

Association to Combat Huntington's Chorea
34a Station Road, Hinckley, Leics., LE10 1AP (Tel: 01455 615 558)

Banstead Mobility Centre
Damson Way, Orchard Hill, Queen Mary's Avenue, Carshalton, Surrey,
SM5 4NR (Tel: 0181 770 1151)

British Epilepsy Association
Anstey House, 40 Hanover Square, Leeds, LS3 1BE (Tel: 0113 243
9393)

British Migraine Association
178a High Road, Byfleet, Weybridge, Surrey, KT14 7ED (Tel: 01932
352468)

British Red Cross
9 Grosvenor Crescent, London, SW1X 7EJ (Tel: 0171 235 5454)

British School of Motoring
Disabled Drivers Assessment Units, 81–87 Hartfield Road, London,
SW19 3TJ (Tel: 0181 540 8262)

Disabled Drivers Motor Club
1a Dudley Gardens, London, W13 9LU

Disabled Information Service Westminster
10 Warwick Row, London, SW1E 5EP (Tel: 0171 630 5994)

DVLA
Medical Adviser, Swansea, SA99 1TU (Tel: 01792 783438)

Dyslexia Institute
133 Gresham Road, Staines, TW18 2AJ (Tel: 01784 463851)

Family Support Services for Huntington's Chorea
108 Battersea High Street, London, SW11 3HP (Tel: 0171 223 7000)

Headway (National Head Injuries Association)
200 Mansfield Road, Nottingham, NG1 3HX (Tel: 01602 622382)

Mind National Association for Mental Health
22 Harley Street, London, W1N 2ED (Tel: 0181 519 2122)

Motor Neurone Disease Association
61 Derngate, Northampton, NN1 1UE (Tel: 01604 250505)

Multiple Sclerosis Society of Great Britain and Northern Ireland
25 Effie Road, London, SW6 1EE (Tel: 0171 736 6267)

National Back Pain Association
31–33 Park Road, Teddington, Middlesex, TW11 0AB (Tel: 0181 977 5474)

National Society for Epilepsy
Chalfont St Peter, Gerrards Cross, Buckinghamshire, SL9 0RJ (Tel: 01494 873991)

Parkinson's Disease Society
36 Portland Place, London, W1N 3DG (Tel: 0171 323 1174)

Stroke Association
CHSA House, Whitecross Street, London, EC1Y 8JJ (Tel: 0171 490 7999)

Index